Renal Diseases

Edited by Edward T. Zawada Jr.
and Sohail Abdul Salim

Published in London, United Kingdom

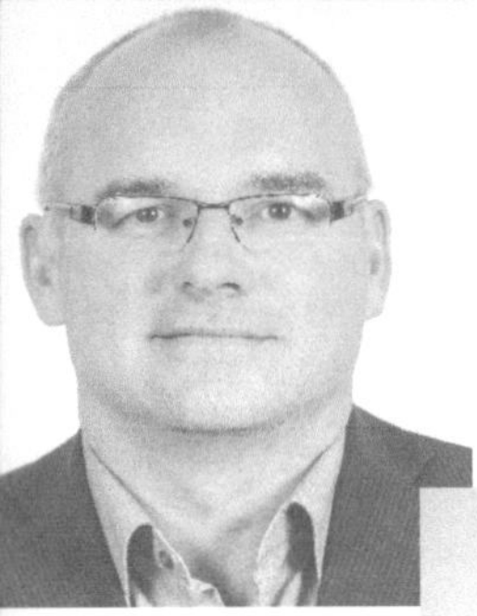
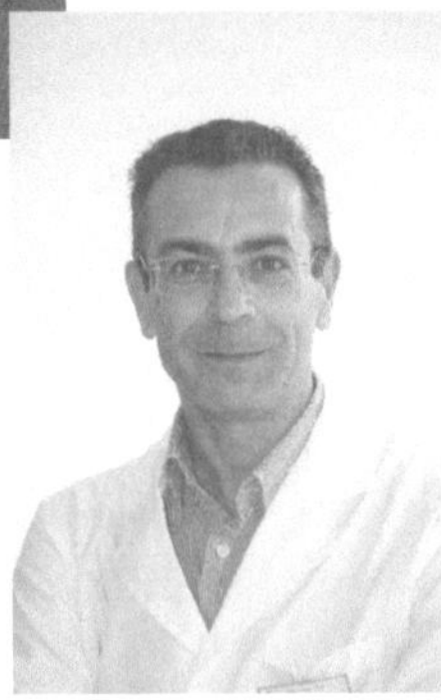
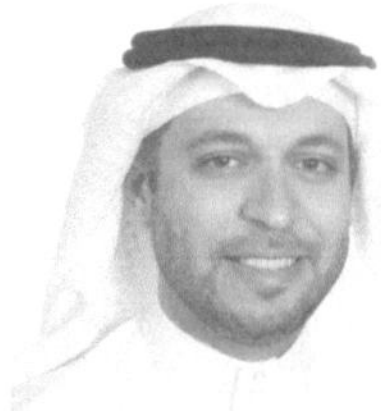
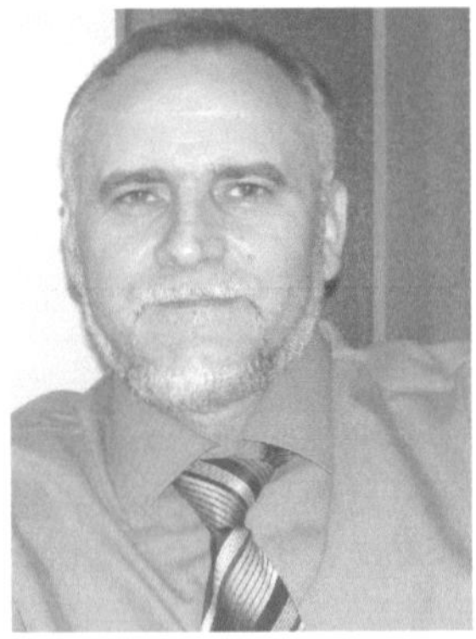
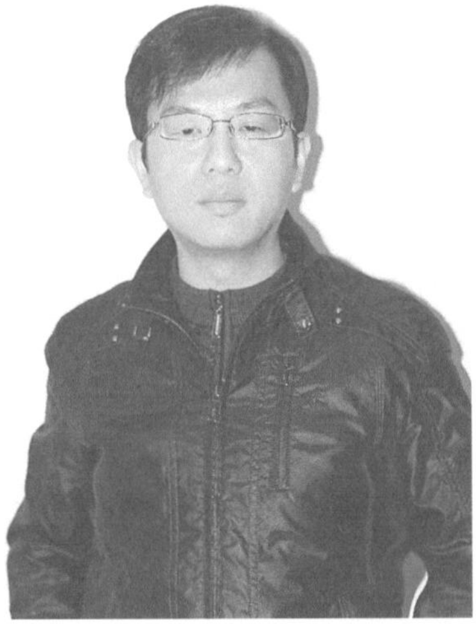
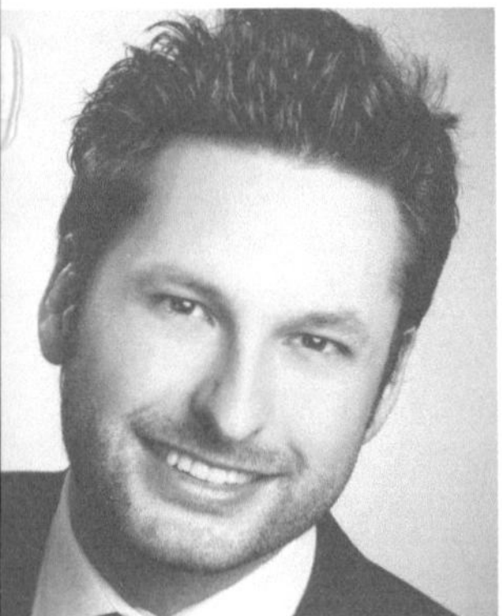
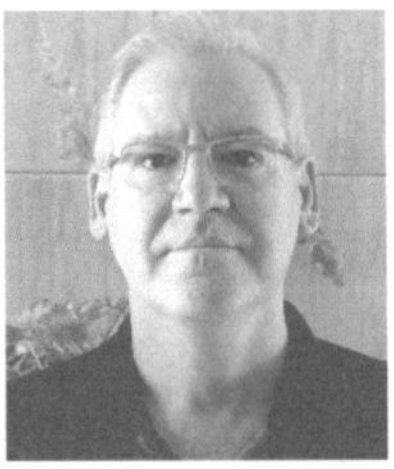

IntechOpen

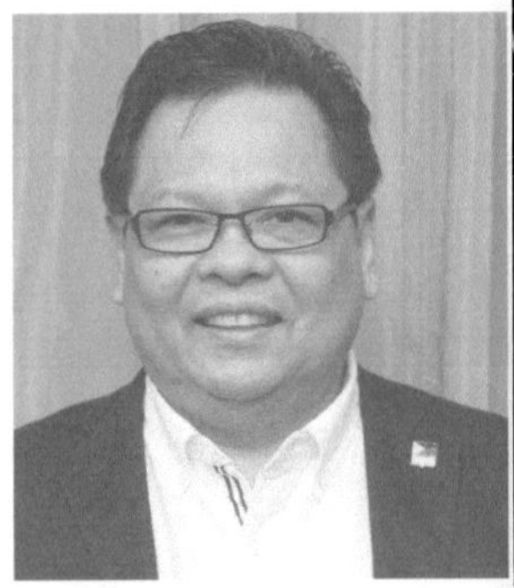
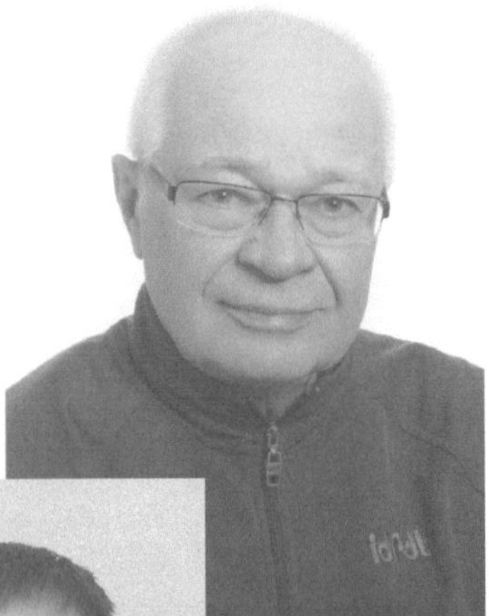
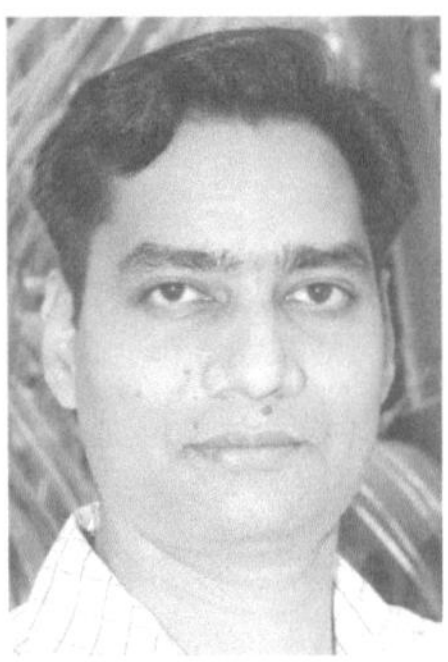
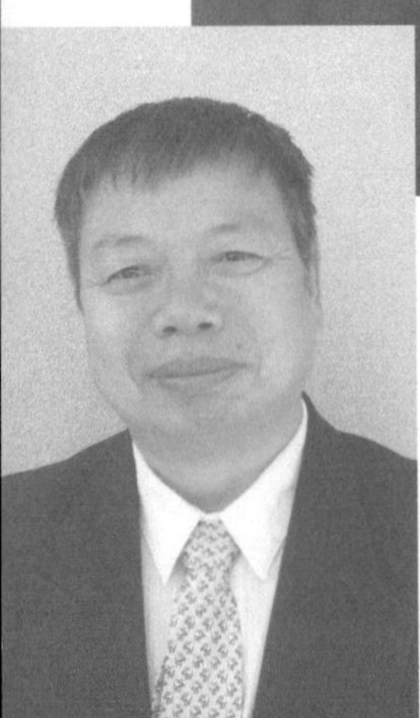
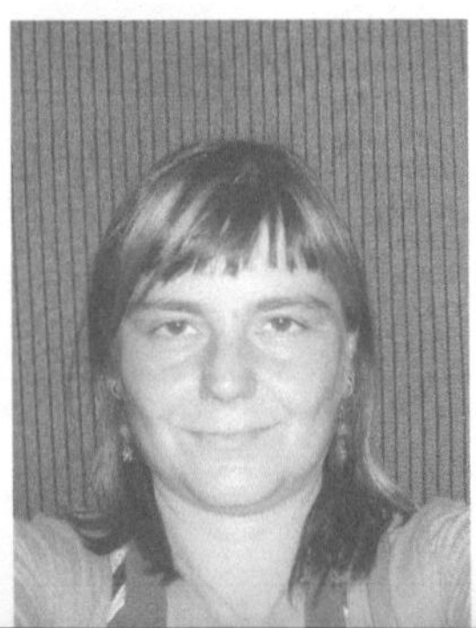
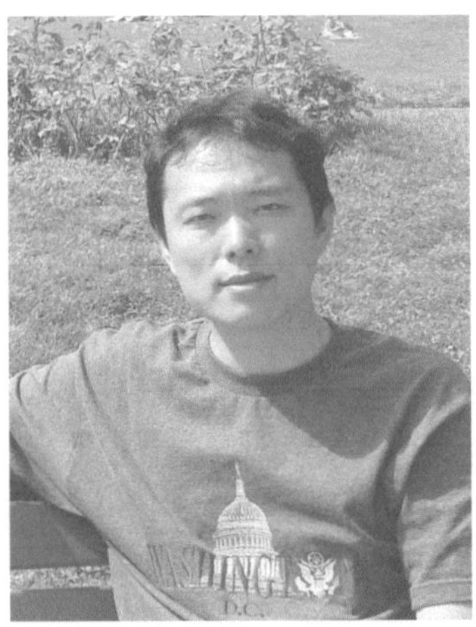

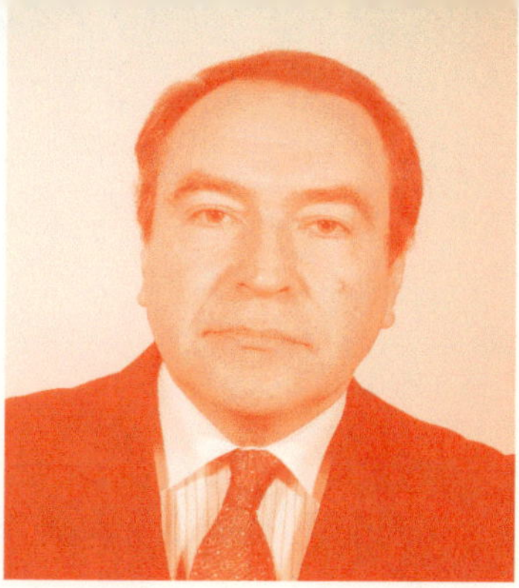
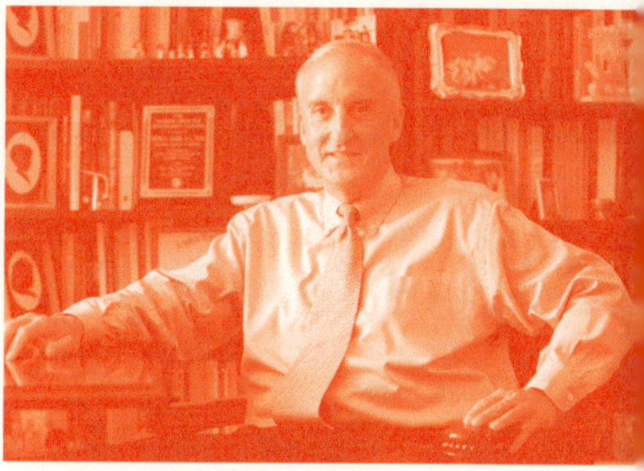
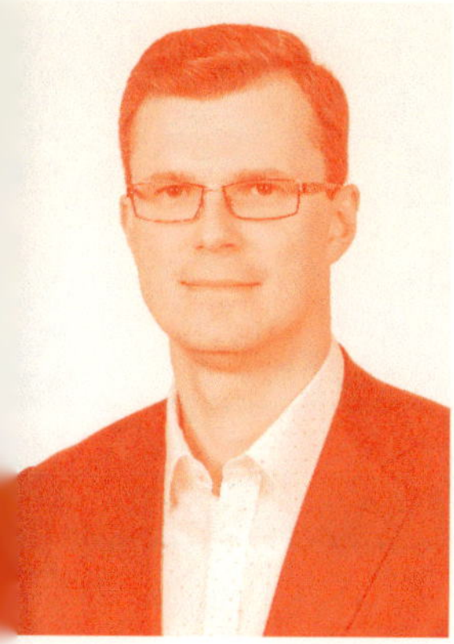
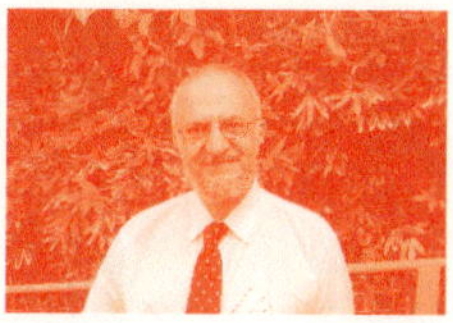
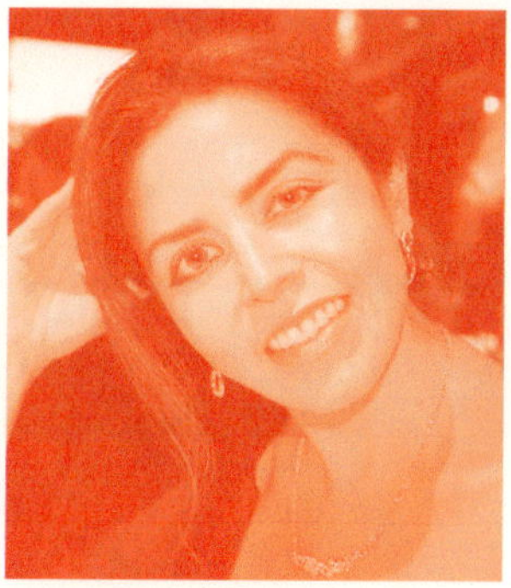

Supporting open minds since 2005

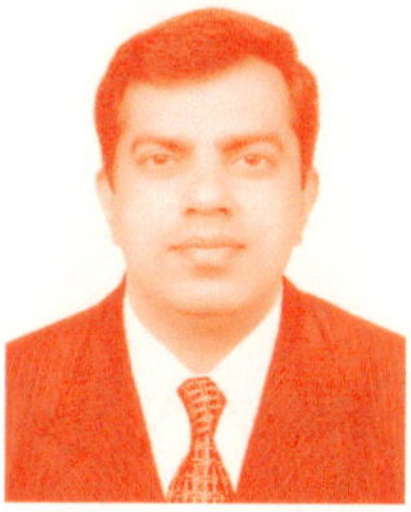
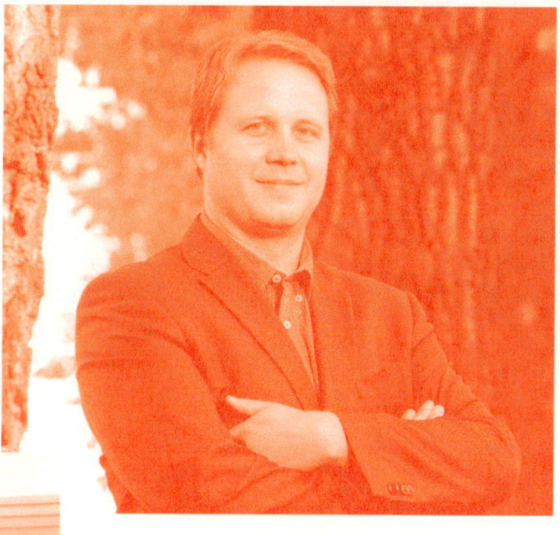
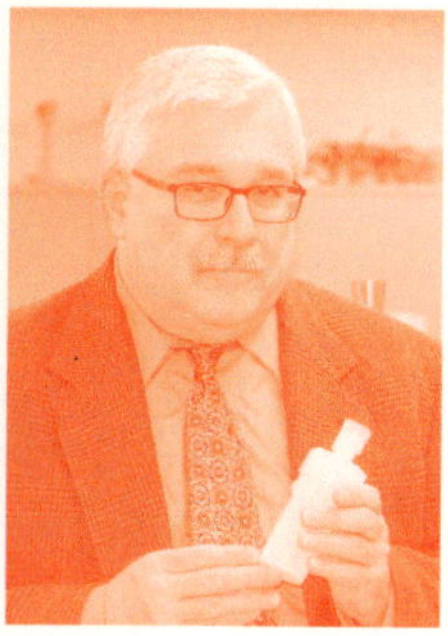
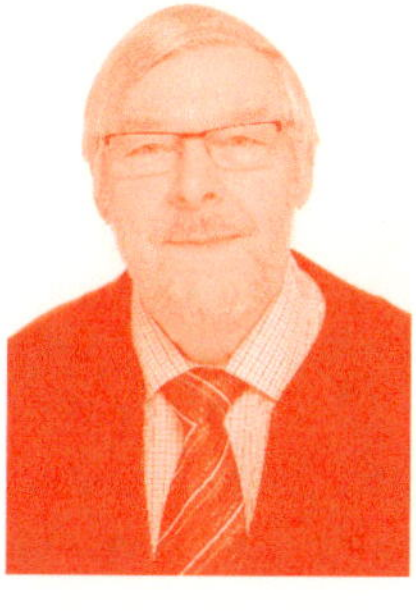
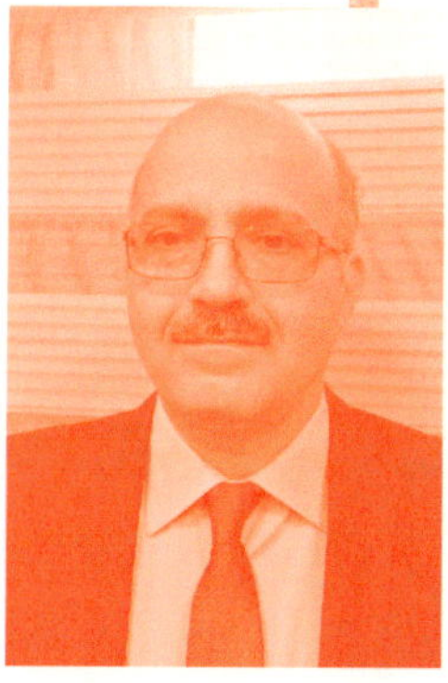
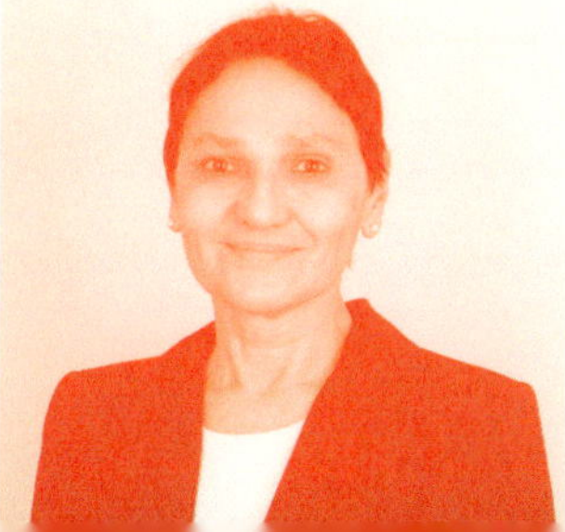
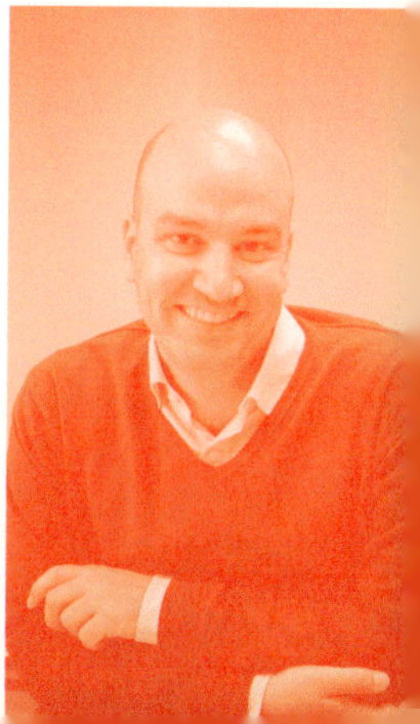

Renal Diseases
http://dx.doi.org/10.5772/intechopen.77765
Edited by Edward T. Zawada Jr. and Sohail Abdul Salim

Contributors
Intezar Ahmed, Enono Yhoshu, Ogochukwu Okoye, Swati Jain, Kirti Jain, Basavaraj Paththi, Maria Carolina Barbosa Álvares, Grupo De Pesquisa Em Radiologia Santa Casa Bh, Fabricio Tinôco Alvim De Souza, Elisa Carvalho De Siqueira, Paulo Ramos Botelho Antunes, Fabiano Franco Monteiro Prado, Luiz Felipe França Antunes, Silvana Maria Carvalho Miranda, Stanley Araujo, Nagaraju Vallepu, Saikiran Velpula, Manishkumar Thimmaraju, Sridhar Babu Gummadi, Bharathkumar Dasari, Edward T. Zawada Jr.

First published in London, United Kingdom, 2020 by IntechOpen
IntechOpen is the global imprint of INTECHOPEN LIMITED, registered in England and Wales, registration number: 11086078, 7th floor, 10 Lower Thames Street, London, EC3R 6AF, United Kingdom
Printed in Croatia

British Library Cataloguing-in-Publication Data
A catalogue record for this book is available from the British Library

Additional hard and PDF copies can be obtained from orders@intechopen.com

Renal Diseases
Edited by Edward T. Zawada Jr. and Sohail Abdul Salim
p. cm.
Print ISBN 978-1-78985-131-1
Online ISBN 978-1-78985-132-8
eBook (PDF) ISBN 978-1-78985-913-3

Meet the editors

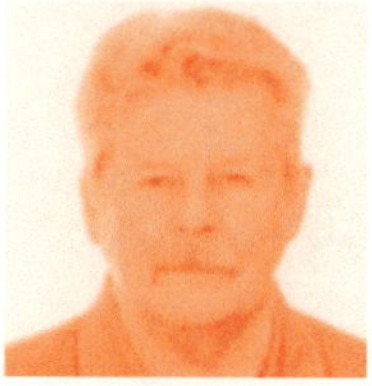

Edward T. Zawada Jr., MD, was born in Chicago, Illinois, in 1947. He graduated summa cum laude with a Bachelor of Science from Loyola University, Chicago, in 1969 and an MD (also summa cum laude) from the Loyola Stritch School of Medicine in 1973. He was inducted into Alpha Omega Alpha in 1972. He trained in internal medicine and nephrology at the David Geffen School of Medicine at UCLA where he later served as an assistant professor of medicine. He had a long career in academic medicine at the University of Utah, Medical College of Virginia, and Sanford School of Medicine of the University of South Dakota where he is a professor and chairman emeritus of the Department of Internal Medicine. He is board certified by the American Board of Internal Medicine in internal medicine, nephrology, geriatrics, and critical care medicine. He also has board certifications in nutrition from the American College of Nutrition, pharmacology by the American Society of Clinical Pharmacology, and hypertension by the American Society of Hypertension. Dr. Zawada has been awarded with fellowship status by the American College of Physicians, the American College of Chest Physicians, the American Heart Association, the American Society of Nephrology, the American Geriatrics Society, the American College of Clinical Pharmacology, the Society for Vascular Medicine, and the Society of Critical Care Medicine. He was also awarded a distinguished service award by the South Dakota Medical Society in 2002 for a career devoted to medical education and master of the American College of Physicians in 2005.

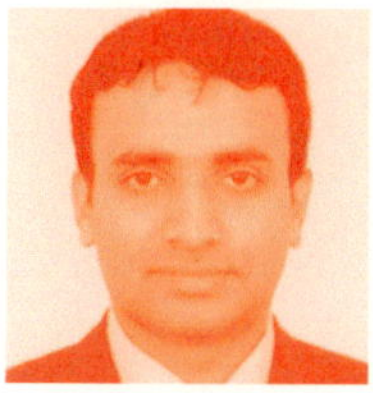

Dr. Sohail Abdul Salim is an American Board Certified Nephrologist practicing in Jackson, Mississippi. He finished his internal medicine residency in 2011 at Brookdale Hospital Medical Center and fellowship in nephrology and hypertension in 2017 from the University of Mississippi. He received a best abstract award from the University of Mississippi and a fellow scholarship from the annual dialysis conference. During the last three years he has authored around ten poster presentations, twenty-seven peer-reviewed publications (most of them as first author) and two book chapters. He has also lectured for multiple conferences, the most recent being "Nephrology Essentials" for the Society of Hospital Medicine. Dr. Salim serves as a reviewer for at least five journals. His research interests are mostly related to nephrotoxic drugs affecting the kidney and the implications in clinical practice.

Contents

Preface

I have been practicing nephrology for forty-five years. During this time the incidence and prevalence of diseases that can result in advanced renal failure has steadily increased. Fortunately, simultaneous advances in dialysis and transplantation have kept pace to allow prolonged life support with dialysis or a "second chance" after successful transplantation. Renal diseases are often difficult to manage because they can be explosive and require early intervention. There is often "no going back" to baseline, only stabilization – the sooner the better.

Renal diseases are not as common as other medical problems in outpatient practice. Primary care providers may not have been exposed to these explosive or silent problems during their training. This collection of reports attempts to serve as insight on the types of renal diseases that can cause permanent damage. Included are reports from different authors from around the world to emphasize specific and accurate diagnosis of these diseases by renal biopsy. These reports describe the various techniques available to make the benefits outweigh risk. These techniques result in a quick, same-day, outpatient procedure to get the diagnosis to allow specific treatment.

Renal diseases are often difficult to distinguish from each other when first trying to understand their pathophysiology. The result is inability to tailor therapy to an individual patient without exact diagnosis. Renal biopsy allows for the determination of which vital renal structure is being attacked: glomeruli, tubules, interstitium, or vasculature. Renal biopsy demonstrates what part of the glomeruli is affected, which immune mechanism is causing the pathophysiology, and the percent of glomeruli that have become totally obsolescent due to the disease processes. Renal biopsy by real-time ultrasound has never been safer. It is a vital tool necessary to obtain the initial diagnosis, but also repeat biopsy may be necessary to follow the progress of therapy. Finally, in renal transplant patients who have been given a "second chance", renal biopsy allows for detection of rejection even before clinical or common laboratory tests reveal its presence to allow early and effective intervention and control.

Edward T. Zawada Jr. M.D. M.A.C.P.
Professor and Chairman Emeritus,
Department of Internal Medicina,
University of South Dakota,
Sanford School of Medicine,
Sioux Falls, South Dakota

Nephrologist and Intensivist,
Shasta Critical,
Care Specialists,
Redding, California

Sohail Abdul Salim
Affiliate Faculty,
Division of Nephrology,
University of Mississippi Medical Center,
Jackson, Mississippi

Chapter 1

Introductory Chapter: Renal Diseases

Edward T. Zawada

1. Introduction

Renal diseases are notoriously silent. Renal diseases are notoriously expensive once they have led to end-stage renal failure requiring dialysis or transplantation. Most acute and chronic renal diseases present with rising serum creatinine and blood urea nitrogen, electrolyte abnormalities, frequent proteinuria, occasional red blood cells in the urine, occasional white blood cells in the urine, or renal cells in the urine often mistaken for white blood cells. It is not easy to make a specific diagnosis from these similar presentations.

I will now present the rationale for renal biopsy to establish renal diagnoses [1]. The classification which follows is the opinion of the author and editor based on over 45 years of experience and exposure to the pioneers in use of renal biopsy for diagnosis [2–4]. My goal is to simplify this argument for performing this invasive procedure to clarify the confusing array of renal diseases with indistinct or asymptomatic presentations.

2. Renal disease diagnosis

Acute renal diseases are described as prerenal, renal, and postrenal, but most patients totally recover normal or near-normal renal function. It is the chronic, often symptomless chronic diseases which lead surreptitiously to end-stage renal disease. Chronic diseases include vascular, glomerular, tubular, and interstitial diseases. The main structures of the kidney are arteries and veins, glomeruli, tubules, and interstitium. Renal biopsy is often required to determine the site of injury. As described below, even when the site of injury is known, such as in glomerular diseases, the renal biopsy is needed to distinguish between the many similar diseases in order to develop possible remission-inducing therapy strategies.

I have been teaching about renal diseases since for 40 years since 1979. I have been struck by three main perspectives. First, diseases can occur in very small areas of the structures of the kidney while the rest of the kidney tissues work well and try to compensate. Second, glomerular diseases are confusing to understand because one needs a framework to separate the multiple very similar diseases into separate clinically relevant entities allowing individual management. Finally, the tubular diseases are the most silent of renal diseases, needing more effort to teach, understand, identify, and manage. Renal biopsy results will be briefly described as the tool to make a definitive diagnosis necessary for proper patient management.

IntechOpen

3. Renal biopsy

Normal renal histology must be known to the clinician before biopsy can be interpreted. The glomeruli will be numerous and have wide-open, thin-walled capillary loops; no inflammatory cells seen; and no increase in numbers of mesangial cells. There can be less than 30% of any glomerulus or all glomeruli which contain amorphous loss of architecture called sclerosis. The blood vessels need to be open without cellular or muscular thickening. Finally, the cross section of renal tubules normally abuts directly against each other without evidence of inflammatory cells or scarring by fibrosis between them.

4. Renal diseases identified by biopsy

Glomerular diseases require the visualization of light microscopy to best understand the numerous entities, many of which have similar immune-mediated pathophysiology. There are nine main light microscopic patterns. Each has a primary and secondary form. This classification allows one to understand the differences of 18 different confusing entities. These patterns are nil lesion, diffuse membranous, diffuse proliferative, diffuse membranoproliferative, focal proliferative, focal sclerosis, nodular glomerulosclerosis, fibrillary, and amyloidosis. For almost everyone, there is a primary and secondary form. The primary forms are idiopathic. The secondary forms are due to a bacteria or virus, a drug, or a systemic disease such as lupus. Based on the light microscopy, the clinician determines if there is a definite cause or whether it is primary. From either category a specific management has reached consensus by nephrologists through international symposia and guidelines.

Tubular diseases do not often show azotemia early. Rather subtle electrolyte findings such as hyperkalemia, hyperuricemia, or non-anion gap metabolic acidosis suggest this category of disease. However, since those disturbances can occur with nonrenal diseases such as gastrointestinal problems, they are not often recognized as early signs of renal damage. Renal biopsy helps distinguish the following most common causes: obstructive or reflux nephropathy, hypertensive injury called acute or chronic nephrosclerosis, drug-induced diseases such as due to analgesics, heavy metal injury such as due to lead, crystal diseases such as urate or oxalate, and unknown causes such as Balkan or other environmental nephritides.

Vascular diseases may occur with or without glomerulonephritis. Fibrinoid necrosis, chronic hypertensive changes of the arteries (nephrosclerosis), and vasculitis are the most common patterns. Fibrinoid necrosis is seen with malignant hypertension, thrombotic thrombocytopenic purpura, scleroderma, eclampsia, and disseminated intravascular coagulation.

Interstitial diseases are identified by acute and chronic inflammatory cells or fibroblasts and collagenous scarring between the tubules causing secondary tubular injury and renal failure. Chronic allograft nephropathy and chronic pyelonephritis are two examples.

5. Conclusion

The above framework to be used for the management of patients with chronic unexplained or understood renal insufficiency is frequently changing. New entities are appearing to add more patterns, more secondary causes of glomerular diseases, and new algorithms for management [5, 6]. Renal disease due to human immunodeficiency virus, new drugs including new biologicals, and new immunologic diseases accounts for some of these newer entities.

In conclusion, a word should be said about repeat renal biopsies. Repeat biopsies are encouraged to assess response to treatment such as in allograft rejection. Repeat biopsies are used to reassess those diseases such as lupus nephritis which can change course leading to new pathophysiology and demanding a change in therapeutic strategy.

Finally, the group at New York Presbyterian/Columbia University Medical Center should be commended as they have continued to provide the most comprehensive annual tutorial and update of the interpretation of renal biopsies based on the very large number of biopsies referred to them [7]. Many of the chapters in this book concentrate on the importance of renal biopsy for diagnosis. Other chapters deal with methods of performing renal biopsy. Finally, there are chapters dealing with complications of renal biopsy.

Author details

Edward T. Zawada
Department of Internal Medicine, Sanford School of Medicine, University of South Dakota, Sioux Falls, United States

*Address all correspondence to: ezawada@sio.midco.net

References

[1] Luiano RL, Moekel GW. Update on the native kidney biosy: Core curriculum 2019. American Journal of Kidney Diseases. 2019;**79**:404-415

[2] Pollak VE, Pirani C, Schwarz FD. The natural history of the renal manifestations of systemic lupus erythematosus. The Journal of Laboratory and Clinical Medicine. 1964; **63**:537-560

[3] Kark RM. The development of percutaneous renal biopsy in man. American Journal of Kidney Diseases. 1990;**XVI**:585-589

[4] Visconti L, Camaro V, Ricciardi CA, Laava V, Pelliano V, Laoquaniti A, et al. Renal biopsy - still a landmark for the nephrologist. World Journal of Nephrology. 2016;**5**(4):321-327

[5] Moutzouris DA, Herlitz L, Appel GB, Markowitz GB, Freudenthal B, Radhkrshman R, et al. Renal biopsy in the very elderly. Clinical Journal of the American Society of Nephrology. 2009; **4**(6):1073-1082

[6] Ramirez G, Saba SR. Primary glomerulonephritis in the elderly. In: Zawada ET Jr, Sica D, editors. Geriatric Nephrology and Urology. Littleton Massahussetts: PSG Publishing Company, Inc.; 1985. pp. 49-66

[7] Hae-Yoon G, Bomback AS, Stokes MB, Santoriello D, Campenot ES, Batal I, et al. The spectrum of kidney biopsy findings in patients with morbid obesity. Kidney International. 2019;**95**: 647-654

Chapter 2

Role of Surgery in Nephrotic Syndrome

Intezar Ahmed and Enono Yhoshu

Abstract

Nephrotic syndrome can occur at any age—adult or children—though the etiology and histopathology may be different in these groups. The management is mostly medical and supportive, but there is some role of surgery in certain complications of nephrotic syndrome, which are rarely discussed together. Here we would like to elaborate some of the areas that require the involvement of surgeons in patients with nephrotic syndrome, to list the complications, and to discuss in brief the surgeries involved. There is a need for randomized prospective studies of nephrotic syndrome patients needing surgical interventions to further project their precise relations and outcomes.

Keywords: surgery, nephrotic syndrome, proteinuria, obesity

1. Introduction

Nephrotic syndrome occurs as a result of pathological injury to the glomeruli of the kidneys. It can be a primary problem, with a disorder which is renal specific or secondary due to a systemic disorder like diabetes mellitus. Consultation of a nephrologist (ideally within 2 weeks) is necessary, and a renal biopsy may need to be performed. This helps in diagnosing what form of glomerular disease is present. More tests may be necessary to rule out secondary disorders, e.g., systemic lupus erythematosus, diabetes mellitus, amyloidosis (AL), etc.

Typically, around 80% of patients remit with oral corticosteroid therapy (steroid sensitive). About 75–85% of these children will have a relapse. Five percent fail to go into remission despite 8 weeks of high-dose steroid therapy and are called as steroid resistant. The primary aim of treatment is to achieve remission, improve symptoms, and prevent, if not at least treat, acute risks such as infection, thrombosis, hypovolemia, etc. On the long term the treating nephrologist's goal should be to prevent complications like high blood pressure, Cushing syndrome, bone disease, obesity, failure to thrive, striae, eye diseases, and a variety of psychological, social, and behavioral disturbances.

The role of surgery in nephrotic syndrome is not directed for patients with primary causes, but only as supportive or symptomatic care. Surgery has some role in nephrotic syndrome patients with secondary etiology, which will be mentioned below separately.

2. Primary causes of nephrotic syndrome requiring surgery

2.1 Infectious complications

An estimate of 17% of infection incidence is observed in nephrotic syndrome patients. Many complications are described in the literature pertaining to the nephrotic

IntechOpen

syndrome such as skin infection, peritonitis, pneumonia, urinary tract infections, bacteremia, etc. Cellulitis is one of the troublesome complications of nephrotic syndrome. The major risk factor for cellulitis is hypoalbuminemia which occurs secondary to proteinuria in these patients [1, 2]. Edema, one of the pathognomonic features of nephrotic syndrome patients, is also credited to hypoalbuminemia as well. The lymphatic flow gets obstructed as a consequence of edema which causes the congregation of bacteria and leads to infection. Abscesses can occur as a consequence of untimely detection and management of cellulitis [3]. Abscesses in nephrotic syndrome have been reported, e.g., subphrenic, perinephric, submandibular, retroperitoneal, and subcutaneous tissues, the brain, and the lung [4]. The adequate drainage of these abscesses anywhere either by open drainage or with percutaneous drainage tubes in conjunction with the appropriate antibiotics is essential for a good outcome.

Out of many, one of the most common infections is bacterial peritonitis found in about 1.4–3.7% of the children and amounting to a mortality rate of 9%. The common bacterial causes of peritonitis have been Gram-positive bacteria, particularly *S. pneumoniae*, but of late Gram-negative bacteria, such as *E. coli*, have been seen to appear. The recommendation for antibiotics has been aminoglycosides and/or third-generation cephalosporins. The controversy regarding the management approaches with laparotomy and laparoscopy exists. Nevertheless, laparoscopic peritoneal washing is sometimes recommended, as it has been shown to decrease the bacterial load in these patients [5].

Studies from India regarding infections in nephrotic syndrome patients by Gulati et al. and Srivastava et al. reported infection rate to be around 32–38% [6, 7]. In spite of the frequent rate of infections in nephrotic syndrome patients as mentioned above, we could not find any literature about the frequency of surgical intervention required for each infective complication, rather, only case reports, probably suggesting the infrequent requirement of surgeries [3, 8]. This could be because of the response of the infections, be it cellulitis or peritonitis of other infections, to adequate and prompt medical supportive measure, including steroids. On the other hand, the fulminant nature of infections in nephrotic syndrome patients if not treated early has been reported.

There is no data to date regarding the wound healing after surgery in nephrotic syndrome patients with cellulitis. Maroz et al. gave a description recently on the relation between the different types of renal impairments and their effects on wound healing [9]. This included acute kidney injury (AKI), chronic kidney disease (CKD), and end-stage renal disease (ESRD) patients and the various implications each has on poor wound healing, but there was no mention of nephrotic patients. Greff et al. in their writing on intra- and postoperative adverse effects of nephrotic syndrome patients needing surgery under general anesthesia reported that in their population of 24 patients, there were no infectious events observed up to 5 days postoperatively [10]. Their population of patients was on long-term antibiotic therapy and was added on specific antibiotics during and after surgeries.

2.2 Dialysis catheter insertion

In the long term, nephrotic syndrome can initiate irreversible kidney injury that further leads to kidney failure and makes treatment with dialysis or, ultimately, kidney transplant essential. Nephrotic syndrome constitutes up to 12% of the causes of end-stage renal disease in children. Dialysis can be of two types—hemodialysis (HD) and peritoneal dialysis [11]. The peritoneal dialysis catheter is usually inserted by a surgeon. For this procedure the abdominal wall is cleaned well in preparation for surgery, and a catheter is inserted surgically with one end in the abdominal cavity and the other outside the body. There are two methods for this procedure to complete open surgery or minimally invasive surgery (laparoscopic). Nowadays, minimally invasive catheter placement technique is an acceptable method. The advantages of minimally invasive/laparoscopic technique are safety, less complications due to entire under vision procedure, less catheter malfunction, prolong catheter life-span, etc. There are well-known important catheter-related complications such as leakage due to tube blockage, infection at entry/exit site and/or tunnel, malposition of catheter tip, hernia, and peritonitis. Of late percutaneous catheter placement technique also emerged that can be performed by an interventional radiologist/nephrologist/surgeon to provide a fast, safe, and reliable peritoneal access.

2.3 Arteriovenous fistula creation

Appropriate and efficient vascular access is necessary for a successful HD. According to the National Kidney Foundation Kidney Disease Outcomes Quality Initiative (NKF-KDOQI) guidelines, the ideal vascular access is described as one which can deliver an adequate flow rate along with durability and a low complication rate. An arteriovenous fistula (AVF) is usually considered to be the best access for HD in adults and, as commented on by an emerging body of evidence, that it is the same also in children [12].

It has been seen that children's vascular biology is not the same as that of adults; henceforth, the ideal size of the vein and artery, anastomosis maturation time, and volume flow rates for a functional fistula in children on HD are not known. Since its inception, advances in AVF creation, especially with improved surgical experience, primary failure rates have been gone down to as low as 5%. For an AVF creation, the preferred sites include, in order, the radial artery to cephalic vein (radiocephalic), brachial artery to cephalic vein (brachiocephalic), and brachial artery to basilic vein (brachiobasilic, with or without transposition). Alternatively, an ulnar artery to basilic vein AVF can be created. Though rarely utilized, an AVF between femoral artery to saphenous vein has also been described. Although there are no guidelines regarding ideal/minimum vessel size in the literature, the general consensus is a minimum venous diameter of 2.5 mm. The essential information before AVF creation includes adequate vessel size; venous stenosis/occlusion can be obtained by duplex ultrasound scanning or venography and is necessary to be carried out in children to decide on the best vessels for AVF creation [13]. Complications of AVF creation include stenosis/occlusion, thrombosis, steal syndrome, and possible discrepancy in limb length if the AVF is placed in the lower extremity. Time for anastomosis maturation may be prolonged, with reports of up to 6 months.

2.4 Renal transplantation

The ultimate treatment for pediatric patients with end-stage kidney disease, including that occurring as a consequence of nephrotic syndrome in the first year of life (NSFL), is renal transplantation. In the early years of renal transplantation era, the results were inferior in young children compared with older children or adults, but in the last few years, results have been improved tremendously mainly because its practice has substantially fine-tuned [14]. Chronic graft loss and opportunistic infectious complications can exist in spite of the improvement in immunosuppression demonstrating excellent results and leading to more 1-year graft survival rates. ESRD in children and adolescents is different from the adult population, in terms of the need to thrive well or have normal growth and have cognitive, psychological, social, and behavioral development. Therefore, the experience gained from adults cannot be extrapolated to pediatric population [15].

Preemptive transplantation (PET), which signifies transplantation prior to the initiation of dialysis, has recently been introduced in the pediatric population, as it is observed that children undergoing renal transplantation before the features of severe uremia sets in are helped by the avoidance of many of the associated long-term complications of ESRD and dialysis.

One of the common causes of ESRD is focal segmental glomerulosclerosis (FSGS). In idiopathic nephrotic syndrome, FSGS is a common pathologic diagnosis, especially in steroid-resistant cases. After kidney transplantation FSGS is known to recur and frequently followed by graft loss [16].

In renal transplantation, patient size and age matching are generally not essential. In fact, it was seen that there is very high rate of graft loss if one matches very young donors to very young recipients, as a consequence of thrombosis. Hence, now pediatric programs are considering the transplant of adult kidneys into small children, once the recipient attains a sufficient size, typically 6.5–10.0 kg of body weight. It has been seen that the peritoneal cavity of an infant has enough space to accommodate an adult kidney without fear of the compression of graft. It has been observed that if body weight of a child is more than 30 kg, the surgical procedure for a kidney transplantation will be similar to that in an adult. However, if the body weight is less than 10 kg, a midline longitudinal abdominal incision is required, and blood vessels from the donor are connected to the recipient's aorta and inferior vena cava. But a tailored approach is needed in children with a body weight of 10–30 kg, in terms of incision site/size, anastomoses of vessels, and allograft sites on the basis of the child's anatomy [17].

3. Secondary causes of nephrotic syndrome requiring surgery

Increasing evidences are available regarding an emerging causal relationship between renal artery stenosis (RAS)/ischemia and the development of nephrotic syndrome. It is well established now that patients with accelerated hypertension used to have proteinuria of nephrotic range. However, it is rarely seen in patients with essential hypertension. Varying degrees of proteinuria are in unilateral RAS patients but normally in around 0.5 g/day. Reduction in this proteinuria is possible with surgical correction of this hemodynamic problem. Various kinds of surgical corrections are reported like nephrectomy, arterial stenosis correction, percutaneous transluminal angioplasty, and stenting. The use of angiotensin-converting enzyme inhibitors (ACE-I) also has shown benefit in minimizing the proteinuria and degrees of hypertension [18].

3.1 Immunoglobulin light chain amyloidosis (AL)

Up to half of all patients presents with renal involvement at the time of diagnosis. About 40% of patients will land up into end-stage renal disease and ultimately will require renal replacement therapy. Management of nephrotic syndrome is difficult and challenging for patients not yet on dialysis. Ablation of natural filtration through medical and/or surgical means has been used to achieve remission from massive proteinuria associated with the nephrotic syndrome. Conservative treatments consist of mercury salt (sodium mercaptomerin), angiotensin II and cyclosporine, and inhibitors of prostaglandin synthesis. Bilateral renal infarction has been used as a substitute to nephrectomy in patients with chronic kidney disease and massive proteinuria. This is carried out by percutaneous route and renal artery embolized using ethanol and irritant coils. Removal of the kidney surgically offers complete relief from proteinuria but carries the risks of complications of an open surgery in severely debilitated patients. Nephrectomy through minimally invasive techniques is a less invasive procedure, even though this procedure also has been used frequently due to the hazards of complications of hypoalbuminemia, hypotension, deranged coagulation profile, and impaired renal function. A novel approach to renal ablation is laparoscopic ligation of both ureters which has been considered by some surgeons for these patients with proteinuria as a disabling refractory complication [19]. The patient will need a long-term hemodialysis after this.

3.2 Bariatric surgery in nephrotic syndrome due to obesity

About 30 years ago, the initial descriptions of nephropathy associated with obesity were published, which were followed by lots of reports of kidney disease in obese subjects without diabetes. Obesity-associated nephrotic syndrome has been described as a glomerulopathy that presents with a variable kind of proteinuria. The mechanisms of renal injury are attributed to the body adapting adversely to the rise in the excretory load, salt retention, and the direct or indirect effects of hyperinsulinemia/insulin resistance and renal lipotoxicity. The most commonly used treatment for nephropathy associated with obesity stresses on the use of antiproteinuric agents, with ACE inhibitors and angiotensin II receptor blockers, which in turn improve sensitivity to insulin and protect the kidneys and cardiovascular system. Bariatric surgery has been accepted as one of the essential procedures for achieving these goals but involves a reasonable risk [20].

Ramirez et al. in their report of two cases of nondiabetic obese patients with FSGS stated that there was an effective reduction of body weight by bariatric surgery and this was successfully accompanied by sustained remission of proteinuria allowing significant reduction or total removal of blockers of the renin-angiotensin system. Huan et al. also reported a case of obesity-related nephropathy and FSGS on renal biopsy. The patient underwent bariatric surgery and attained successful weight reduction with significant decrease in proteinuria and stabilization of renal function [21].

4. Conclusion

The literature on the role of surgery in nephrotic syndrome is scanty, though the association of nephrologists with surgeons has been ongoing. We have tried to enumerate some of the role of surgeons in nephrotic syndrome patients, with some review of the available literature. In order to bring out more specific outcomes of complications of nephrotic syndrome patients being managed surgically, more randomized controlled studies with better documentation of interventions being done is essential and much needed.

Author details

Intezar Ahmed* and Enono Yhoshu
All India Institute of Medical Sciences, Rishikesh, India

*Address all correspondence to: ahmed_intezar@rediffmail.com

References

[1] Wei CC, Yu IW, Lin AW, Tsai A. Occurrence of infection among children with nephrotic syndrome during hospitalization. Asian Pacific Society of Nephrology. 2012;**17**:681-688

[2] Ajayan P, Krishnamurthy S, Biswal N, Mandan J. Clinical spectrum and predictive risk factors of major management in hospitalized children with nephrotic syndrome. Indian Pedtrics. 2013;**50**:779-781

[3] Siregar RS, Daulay KR, Siregar B, Ramayani OR, Eyanoer PC. Cellulitis as complication of nephrotic syndrome in a pediatric patient. IOP Conference Series: Earth and Environmental Science. 2018;**125**:012111. DOI: 10.1088/1755-1315/125/1/012111

[4] Shinde A, Chatterjee R. Peritonitis with bilateral thigh abscess in nephrotic syndrome: An unusual infection. International Journal of Healthcare and Biomedical Research. 2016;**5**:53-56

[5] Lagos L, Valero J. Coexistence of cellulitis and primary peritonitis in a pediatric patient with nephrotic syndrome: A case report. Journal of Pediatric Surgery Case Reports. 2017;**20**:48-50

[6] Gulati S, Kher V, Sharma RK, Gupta A. Steroid response pattern in Indian children with nephrotic syndrome. Acta Paediatrica. 1994;**83**:530-533

[7] Srivastava RN, Mayekar G, Anand R, Choudhry VP, Ghai OP, Tandon HD. Nephrotic syndrome in Indian children. Archives of Disease in Childhood. 1975;**50**:26-30

[8] Kumar KJ, Solbin J, Kumar MJ, Anitha C. Acute pyogenic psoas abscess in a child with. Sri Lanka Journal of Child Health. 2016;**45**:226-228

[9] Maroz N, Simman R. Wound healing in patients with impaired kidney function. Journal of the American College of Clinical Wound Specialists. 2013;**5**:2-7

[10] Greff B, Faivre J, Carli PA, Niaudet P, Orliaguet GA. Intra- and postoperative adverse events in children with nephrotic syndrome requiring surgery under general anesthesia. Paediatric Anaesthesia. 2012;**22**:244-249

[11] Sharma A, Ramanathan R, Posner M, Fisher RA. Pediatric kidney transplantation: A review. Transplant Research and Risk Management. 2013;**5**:21-31

[12] Shroff R, Sterenborg RB, Kuchta A, Arnold A, Thomas N, Stronach L, et al. A dedicated vascular access clinic for children on haemodialysis: Two years' experience. Pediatric Nephrology. 2016;**31**:2337-2344

[13] Chand DH, Valentini RP, Kamil ES. Hemodialysis vascular access options in pediatrics: Considerations for patients and practitioners. Pediatric Nephrology. 2009;**24**:1121-1128

[14] Mejía SM, Melgar AA, Hijosa MM, Camblor CF, Carrión AP, Meseguer CG, et al. Renal transplantation in children with nephrotic syndrome in the first year of life. Transplantation Proceedings. 2015;**47**:38-41

[15] Saeed B. Pediatric renal transplantation. International Journal of Organ Transplantation Medicine. 2012;**3**:62-73

[16] Kang HG, Ha IS, Cheong HI. Recurrence and treatment after renal transplantation in children with FSGS. BioMed Research International. 2016;**2016**:1-7

[17] Dharnidharka VR, Fiorina P, Harmon WE. Kidney transplantation in

children. The New England Journal of Medicine. 2014;**371**:549-558

[18] Bhandari S, Kalowski S. Surgical correction of nephrotic syndrome. Nephron. 2001;**87**:291-292

[19] Keddis MT, Stegall MD, Textor SC. Renal ablation using bilateral ureteral ligation for nephrotic syndrome due to renal amyloidosis. Clinical Kidney Journal. 2012;**5**:153-154

[20] Ramírez J, Carpio D, Mezzano S, Mukdsi J, Ardiles L. Bariatric surgery in patients with focal segmental glomerulosclerosis secondary to obesity. Nefrología. 2009;**29**:266-269

[21] Huan Y, Tomaszewski JE, Cohen DL. Resolution of nephrotic syndrome after successful bariatric surgery in patient with biopsy-proven FSGS. Clinical Nephrology. 2009;**71**:69-73

Chapter 3

Renal Biopsy: Appraisal of the Methods

Ogochukwu Okoye

Abstract

Renal biopsy is an invasive specialized test aimed at obtaining renal tissue for histologic diagnosis of a variety of kidney diseases. Common indications for renal biopsy in practice include adult nephrotic syndrome, steroid resistant or clinically atypical nephrotic syndrome in children, glomerulonephritis, acute kidney injury (AKI) of unknown aetiology, systemic diseases with renal involvement, and persistent proteinuria or haematuria with reduced renal function. Over the years there has been continuous refinement of renal biopsy techniques. It is now mostly performed percutaneously using imaging guidance and more sophisticated spring-loaded needles of varying sizes. Other non-percutaneous techniques such as transjugular, laparoscopic and open renal biopsy are also being performed especially in patients with contraindications to the percutaneous approach. Percutaneous ultrasound guided approach is standard care for biopsy of non-focal lesions. The CT-guided method can be used in obese patients and other patients who are unable to lay prone, patients with complex anatomy, and when the kidneys are not sufficiently visualised by ultrasound scan. The transjugular technique is most popular for combined liver and kidney biopsy. The major advantages of the laparoscopic and open biopsy techniques are the opportunity for direct visualization of the kidney and good intra-operative haemostasis.

Keywords: renal biopsy, transjugular biopsy, percutaneous renal biopsy, open renal biopsy

1. Introduction

Renal biopsy is an invasive specialized test aimed at obtaining renal tissue for histologic diagnosis of a variety of kidney diseases. Kidney biopsy is generally indicated when, (1) the cause of kidney disease cannot be sufficiently determined or predicted clinically or by less invasive diagnostic procedures, (2) clinical features suggest parenchymal disease that can be diagnosed by pathologic evaluation and (3) the differential diagnosis includes diseases that have different treatments, prognosis or both [1].

Common indications for renal biopsy in practice include adult nephrotic syndrome, steroid resistant or clinically atypical nephrotic syndrome in children, glomerulonephritis, acute kidney injury (AKI) of unknown aetiology, systemic diseases with renal involvement, and persistent proteinuria or haematuria with reduced renal function. Sometimes diagnosis of kidney disease is clinically apparent, however a biopsy may be required for confirming diagnosis, assessing disease activity, chronicity and severity, e.g. in systemic lupus erythematosus [2].

Renal biopsy may be associated with complications such as bleeding, pain, infections, injury to contiguous structures, and very rarely loss of a kidney or death of the patient. The safety and usefulness of renal biopsy in the diagnosis, monitoring and treatment of renal parenchymal diseases largely depends upon correct selection and adequate preparation of the patient, the skillfulness of the operator, and the technique used.

Over the years there has been a continuous refinement of renal biopsy techniques. It is mostly performed percutaneously using imaging guidance and more sophisticated soft-tissue needles (**Figure 1a-c**) of varying sizes. Other

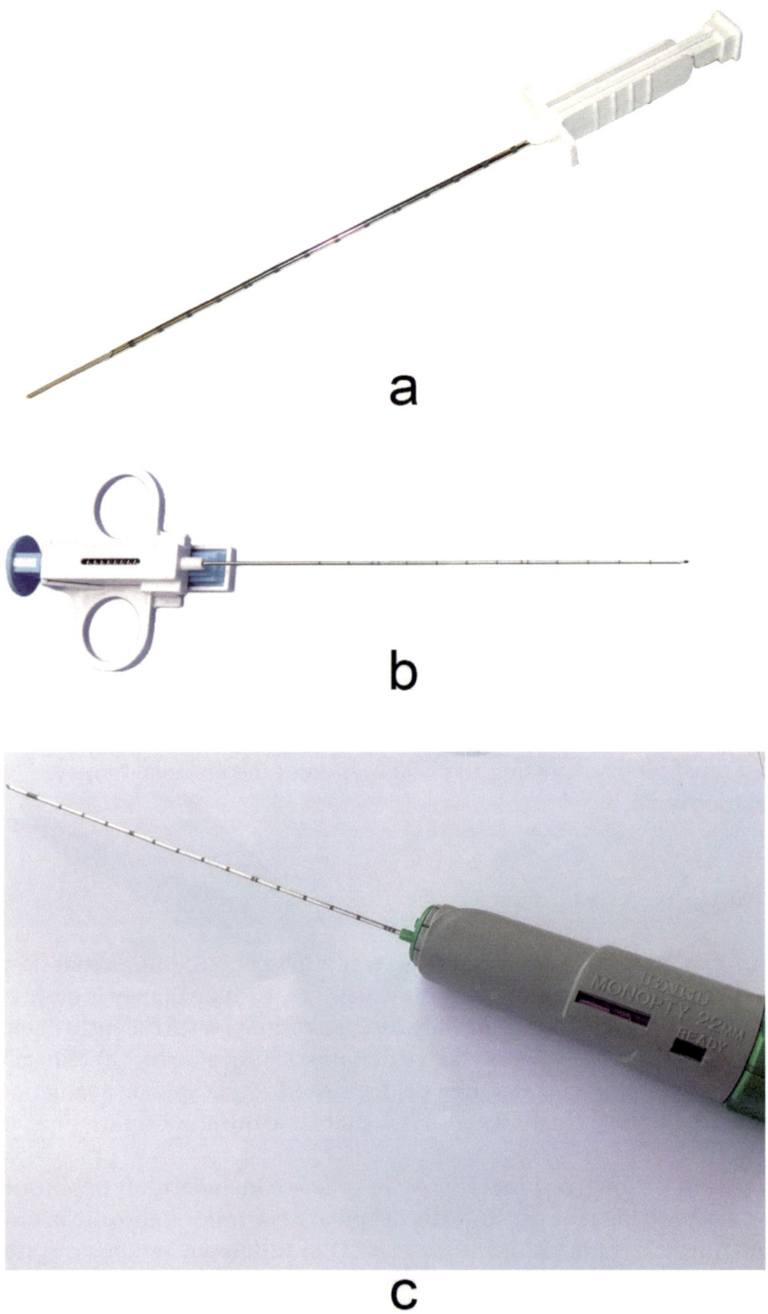

Figure 1.
Soft tissue biopsy needles: (a) Tru-Cut, (b) semi-automated biopsy needle, and (c) automated biopsy needle.

non-percutaneous techniques such as transjugular renal biopsy, laparoscopic and open renal biopsy are also being performed especially in patients with contraindications to the percutaneous approach.

2. Methods of renal biopsy

Iversen and Brun introduced percutaneous renal biopsy (PRB) of native kidneys in 1951, when they performed the procedure in a sitting patient using an aspiration needle after localizing the kidney with intravenous pyelography [3]. Although this innovation revolutionized the nephrology practice at the time, the tissue yield was inadequate in up 47% of the biopsies they performed over time [3]. Since then other percutaneous methods have been introduced and practiced with better tissue yields of up to 95–99% in some series [4–6]. Despite these encouraging figures, the tissue obtained is sometimes not diagnostically useful. This can be due to poor patient selection, wrong or poor technique, and inappropriate tissue handling, i.e., division of tissue for the different histopathologic examinations, and storage. The nephrologist should be adequately knowledgeable of indications, contraindications and complications of renal biopsy, and the several techniques available. This will significantly help to improve the usefulness of this procedure in terms of individual patient care and outcome.

Renal biopsy may be performed by one of the following approaches: percutaneous blind, blind after localisation with ultrasound scan, percutaneous real-time ultrasound guided, percutaneous CT guided, transjugular renal biopsy, laparoscopic renal biopsy, and open renal biopsy. The choice of technique among physicians often depends on skillfulness, availability of equipment and compelling indications in the patient. The techniques are briefly described below.

2.1 Percutaneous blind

This technique is now obsolete in advanced countries, but still being practiced in some centres in low and low-middle income countries. The patient is placed in the prone position with a pillow or towel under the abdomen; the lower pole of the kidney to be biopsied is localised using the anatomic landmark (the tip of the twelfth rib posteriorly). Thereafter the skin is prepped, draped, and local anaesthetic is used to infiltrate the skin down to the kidneys. Either the manual (Tru-Cut) or spring-loaded biopsy needle is inserted through a nick made on the anaesthetized skin, and advanced towards the renal capsule while patient breaths gently. When the needle just pierces the renal capsule (signified by a give and swinging of the biopsy needle with respiratory excursions), the patient is instructed to hold the breath, and the biopsy cut is taken. Patient is observed usually for at least 6–8 hours, but may require longer admission depending on the presence of complications. This technique can be cumbersome and potentially associated with complications; tissue yield is often not optimal and several passes may be required to obtain adequate tissue.

2.2 Percutaneous ultrasound guided

Percutaneous ultrasound guided biopsy is the standard of care [7]. This technique can be performed blind after localizing the kidney with an ultrasound probe, or performed with real-time ultrasound guidance. The patient is placed in a prone position with a towel or pillow beneath the abdomen to ensure proper positioning and to stabilize the kidney. The lower pole of the kidney is localized using the ultrasound probe placed around the renal angle posteriorly (**Figure 2**). The area of skin overlying the lower pole can be marked and the probe removed (blind) or the probe is used to guide the biopsy needle throughout the procedure (real-time). From this point on the procedure is similar to the blind technique.

The use of ultrasound guidance is now universally available in most countries globally, except for some centres in low and low-middle income countries where the ultrasound machine may not be available in the centre or to the nephrologist. The implication of this is that nephrologists in such centres may not have the skill required and this contributes to declining practice of renal biopsy in many of such centres.

2.3 CT guided percutaneous

CT guided PRB may be the primary imaging technique or is indicated in obese patients, patients with complex kidney anatomy (e.g. vascular anomaly, horse-shoe kidney), focal lesions, those in whom kidneys are not well visualized on ultrasound and in patients who have difficulty lying prone [7, 8]. Interventional nephrologists or radiologists perform this procedure in the CT suite. Patients are usually fasted for 8 hours to allow for administration of conscious sedation. An intravenous line is secured for fluid administration and monitoring equipment for vital signs and pulse oximetry are attached to patient [9]. Patient with difficulties lying prone are placed in the ipsilateral side-up position, however the location of a focal lesion also influences the position chosen, e.g. lesions along the lateral edge of the kidney may be difficult to access with an ipsilateral side-up approach [9].

After adequately positioning the patient, a localizing grid is placed and preliminary CT images at 5 mm axial slices covering the entire length of the kidney is obtained. Thereafter, the shortest and safe route is chosen, the skin overlying kidney is prepped, draped and anaesthetized with 1% lidocaine. A coaxial needle is advanced to the kidney with CT guidance and core biopsy samples or fine needle aspirates are collected [9]. Once all samples are collected the needle is removed and post-care is given, including a post-procedure imaging to exclude haemorrhage.

2.4 Transjugular renal biopsy

Mal who intended to carry out a liver biopsy but accidentally also obtained renal tissue first performed this procedure in 1989 [10]. Thereafter he further explored the feasibility of the procedure and it has since been practiced with success. Transjugular renal biopsy (TJRB) is performed in a radiology suite by either an interventional nephrologist or radiologist with fluoroscopy guidance.

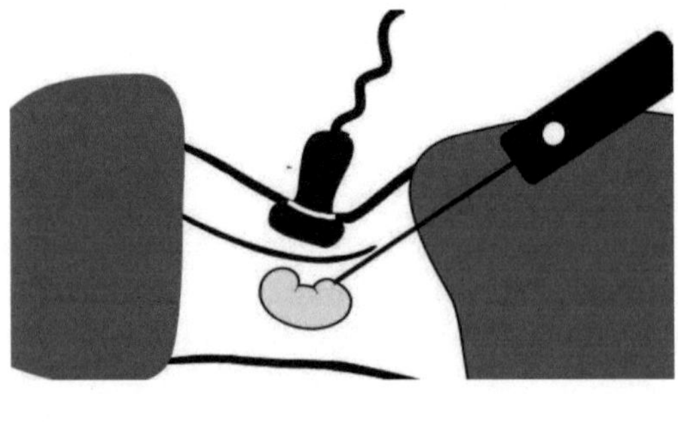

Figure 2.
Percutaneous ultrasound guided renal biopsy.

	US-guided biopsy	CT guided biopsy	Laporoscopic	Open biopsy	Transjugular biopsy
Compelling indications	None	Obese Complex anatomy Focal lesions Poor USS visualization	Obese Complex anatomy Bleeding diathesis Poor visualization Failed PRB Solitary kidney Cystic kidneys High kidney location	Obese Complex anatomy Bleeding diathesis Poor visualization Failed PRB Solitary kidney Cystic kidneys High kidney location	Morbidly obese Bleeding diathesis Liver + kidney biopsy
Contraindications	Hypertension Obesity Small kidneys Bleeding diathesis Solitary kidney Infection Obstructed kidney	History of allergic reaction to contrast	*	Religious grounds	History of allergic reaction to contrast
Tissue yield	Good	Excellent	Excellent	Excellent, abundant	Good
Routine admission required	No	No	Yes	Yes	Yes
Complications	Pain Bleeding Injury to structures Infections	Pain Bleeding Injury to structures Infections Radiation contrast nephropathy	Surgical risks	Surgical risks	Capsular perforation Contrast nephropathy
Skill requirement	+	++	+++	+++	++
G. A	No	No	Yes	Yes	No
Cost	+	++	+++	+++	++

Patient's refusal or uncooperative patients are universal contraindication to all approaches.

Table 1.
Comparing the biopsy techniques.

The aspiration needle or core biopsy approach may be used and the main difference between the two approaches is the biopsy instrument.

The right internal jugular vein is often preferred due to its straighter course to the inferior vena cava. Following injection of local anaesthetic to skin and subcutaneous area, the vein is punctured with an 18-guage needle just above the thyroid cartilage medial to the sternal head of the sternocleidomastoid [11]. A guide wire is inserted and then a venous sheath is introduced over it. Next the catheter is advanced under fluoroscopic guidance through the IVC into the right renal vein. Lastly, the TRJB needle, pre-filled with normal saline and attached to a 20 ml luer lock syringe, is advanced down the catheter to obtain the tissue core (core biopsy technique) [11]. More than one pass is usually possible to improve tissue yield.

2.5 Laparoscopic and open biopsy

Laparoscopic biopsy is usually performed by a urologist mostly via the retroperitoneal approach but can be approached transperitoneally. The patient receives general anaesthesia, is placed in full right or left flank position, prepped and draped. Using a two-port technique, firstly the retroperitoneum is entered in the posterior axillary line, halfway between the ribs and iliac crest [12]. The lower pole of the kidney is then localized by blunt dissection with the laparoscopic lens to create a space posterior to the kidney. Next a 5 mm trochar is inserted under direct vision in the anterior axillary line at the level of the iliac crest to identify the kidney; the biopsy is taken using a laparoscopic biopsy forceps [12]. Multiple biopsies can be taken and thereafter haemostasis is secured. In uncertain cases, intraoperative ultrasonography can be performed via a laparoscopic probe, to confirm renal tissue before biopsy [12, 13].

Open biopsies can be performed in patients with contraindication to PRB, or during open abdominal surgeries for other renal indications, e.g. taking a biopsy during a partial nephrectomy. Some patients refuse open biopsies on religious grounds (Jehovah's witness refusing blood transfusion) [12], so the laparoscopic technique becomes the preferred option (**Table 1**).

3. Specimen handling and processing

The manner in which the biopsy core collected is handled and processed contributes to the diagnostic and prognostic usefulness. The tissue core should be gently removed from the biopsy needle using an 18G needle, or washed from the needle onto a Petri dish, using a slow jet of normal saline. A magnifying lens or a dissecting microscope should be used immediately to confirm it is kidney tissue, and whether it is cortex or medulla. The renal cortex appears pale pink to tan with reddish blushes depicting the glomeruli, while the medulla usually contains straight red striations representing vasa recta [14].

The biopsy operator must be knowledgeable of effective ways of dividing the renal core obtained when needed, and the right fixative to use. This ensures that adequate samples are delivered to the pathologist, for the different processing and fixation methods required for light microscopy (LM), immunohistochemistry (IHC) and electron microscopy (EM). At least three cores are required, one each for LM, IHC and EM. The need for dividing tissue core arises if the number of cores obtained is inadequate, e.g. if only one core is obtained, 1 mm cuts are made from both ends for EM, while the remainder is cut in two, the larger of which is used for LM while the other for IHC [14]. Specimen should be placed quickly in appropriate fixatives and accompanied with adequate clinical information to guide the pathologist in interpreting the findings.

3.1 Light microscopy

The fixative for LM is buffered 10% aqueous formaldehyde solution. The tissue is examined using a light microscope which employs focused visible light to magnify objects viewed. Stains are used to enhance characterization of the tissue; common stains are H&E, periodic acid-Schiff (PAS), Silver, and Trichrome. Light microscopy (LM) shows predominantly proliferative lesions, and occasionally membranous features and crescents. It gives limited magnification and so there is often a need for EM and or IHC to avoid missed diagnosis.

3.2 Immunohistochemistry

This includes immunofluorescence (IF) and immunoperoxidase (IP). The choice of which to use often depends on the pathologist and resources available. Immunoperoxidase (IP) requires no special fixation, since a tissue pre-fixed in formalin for LM can be used for IP depending on the question to be answered. It produces well-developed antigen retrieval and results are reproducible [14]. Immunofluorescence is the choice of most renal pathologist. The fixation used is Zeus solution (modified Michel's tissue fixative). IF produces accurate location of deposits with the aid of dark field microscopes, and excellent resolution when fluorescence microscopes with epifluorescence attachments are used. Routine examinations during IF include immunoglobulin's (IgG, IgM, IgA), complements (C3, C1q, C4) fibrin, kappa and lambda chains. Other antibodies may be examined depending on the question to be answered, e.g. C4d in allograft biopsies.

3.3 Electron microscopy

The fixative for EM is 2–3% glutaraldehyde or 1–4% paraformaldehyde. Electron microscopy (EM) aids in visualizing the ultrastructure and cross section of the kidney tissue including the glomerular basement membrane, mesangium, capillary loops, tubulointerstitium, vessels. Immune deposits are also well visualized.

Ideally all three histopathologic examinations discussed above should be performed on all individual patient's specimens received to avoid missed diagnosis. Diagnosis such as light chain-associated disease, IgA nephropathy, anti-glomerular basement membrane disease may be missed without IHC, while diagnosis such as minimal change disease, fibrillary glomerulopathy, immunotactoid glomerulopathy, dense deposit disease, Alports, and thin glomerular basement membrane nephropathy may be missed without an EM.

4. Appraisal of the methods

The image guided percutaneous techniques are successful in terms of tissue yield in majority of cases. Furthermore, image guidance is particularly instrumental to the safe performance of focus biopsies in cases of cystic kidneys and solid renal masses [9]. Apart from methods described earlier, newer imaging techniques, such as, CT fluoroscopy and fusion ultrasonography may apply to renal biopsy in the future [15].

Percutaneous ultrasound guided approach is standard care for biopsy of non-focal lesions [7]. The real-time ultrasound guided technique has been compared to the blind technique after localisation with ultrasound, and no significant difference in tissue yield was noted [16]. Both techniques have similar potential complications and can be used in similar patients. The rates of complications associated with PRB are difficult to compare across studies because of the heterogeneity of studies in terms of technique and needle used, operator and definitions of complications, e.g. bleeding [7]. These procedures are however done routinely without need for overnight admission except severe complications arise.

Tissue diagnosis may not be successful in about 6% of ultrasound guided biopsies in some series and common reasons are due to operator's technique, type/size of biopsy needle, and patient factors (reduced GFR, small atrophic kidneys, anatomically complex kidneys). Some comparative studies have reported that automated needles provide superior yield and lower major complication rates than older, hand-driven (Tru-Cut) systems [17, 18]. A 14- or 16-gauge needle provides larger cores and the tissue yields are comparable however, the 14-gauge needle is reportedly associated with more bleeding complications [19, 20]. The 18-gauge needle on the other hand is smaller and some studies report a lower tissue yield [19, 20]. A study by Kriegshauser et al. found that operator experience, taking multiple specimens, and using the cortical tangential approach significantly improved the pathologic material obtained during native renal biopsies [21]. It also helps to have a light microscope available during renal biopsy procedure, to visualize biopsy core immediately after it is obtained.

The CT-guided method can be used in obese patients and other patients who are unable to lay prone, patients with complex anatomy, and when the kidneys are not sufficiently visualised by ultrasound scan [8]. This procedure has been associated with 100% success in some reports [22]. Biopsy of focal lesions is more successful with CT-guidance using either core biopsy or aspiration needle, although some authors have reported increased diagnostic yield when a combination of both needles are used [9]. Unlike the ultrasound-guided technique, it is not performed real-time and patients are exposed to some radiation. Most patients will usually require conscious sedation but can be discharged a few hours after the procedure provided there are no major complications.

Contraindications to PRB such as uncontrolled severe hypertension, morbid obesity, uncontrolled bleeding diathesis, solitary kidney, small kidneys, complex kidney anatomy (e.g. high location, horse-shoe kidney), and renal impairment; are often reasons for selection of alternative techniques. Additionally, failed percutaneous biopsy, poor visualization on imaging, cystic kidney with rapidly progressing GN, and high location of the kidneys are some indications for a laparoscopic or open biopsy [13]. The major advantages of the laparoscopic and open biopsy techniques are the opportunity for direct visualization of the kidney and good intra-operative haemostatic control of the biopsy site [13]. The tissue yield is often abundant and diagnostically useful, however the risks of general surgery/anaesthesia, need for special surgical skill, overnight admissions and high costs are some of the disadvantages.

The transjugular technique is most popular for combined liver and kidney biopsy, and in patients with certain contraindications to PRB (bleeding, inability to lie prone due to obesity, ascites or respiratory difficulty) in whom pathological diagnosis might alter clinical management. Diagnostic yield is comparable with PRB, but differs slightly depending on the approach used, 73–95% diagnostic yield has been reported for the aspiration needle approach [23–26] compared with 89–96.5% for the core biopsy needle [27, 28]. Although judged to be a safe and efficient procedure, there is the risk of contrast induced nephropathy and capsular perforation, which might require coil embolisation. Major complications are seen in 1–18% of cases when using the aspiration needle [23–26], compared to 2.7–27% with the core biopsy technique [27, 28]. Rathod et al. in India reported capsular perforation in five out of nine patients who had TRJRB using the core biopsy approach, although none had major event requiring intervention (blood transfusion or embolisation) [11]. Contrast nephropathy is a concern given that a significant proportion of patients undergoing this procedure have baseline renal impairment, but only 15–30 ml of contrast is used. There is usually no need for overnight stay as patient can be discharged as early as 4 hours post procedure.

Finally, regardless of the renal biopsy method selected, the nephrologist must ensure adequate pre- and post-care of the patient and obtain informed consent. Biopsy protocols should ideally exist in every centre carrying out renal biopsies, and should be strictly adhered to. It is standard practice before kidney biopsies to check patient's vital signs, obtain a complete blood count, international normalized ratio/prothrombin time, activated partial thromboplastin time, serum creatinine, urine culture, and group/crossmatch blood. Medications should be reviewed for drugs that may increase bleeding risk. Intravenous access is needed and anxious, uncooperative, and/or pediatric patients may require conscious sedation or general anesthesia. Biopsy tissue histology must only be interpreted by experienced and competent pathologists.

5. Conclusion

Renal biopsy can be an indispensable tool in the diagnosis, monitoring, treatment, and prognosis, of patients with non-focal or focal renal parenchymal disease or systemic diseases with renal manifestation. The diagnostic usefulness significantly depends upon the operator's ability to select and prepare the patient based on in depth knowledge of the indications, contraindications and complications. The operator's skill, choice of technique and instruments are key factors that will determine the safety and efficacy of the procedure.

Acknowledgements

H3Africa Kidney Research Network, for providing my division with training and equipment support for percutaneous ultrasound guided renal biopsy.

Conflict of interest

The author declares no conflict of interest.

Author details

Ogochukwu Okoye
Department of Internal Medicine, Delta State University, Abraka, Nigeria

*Address all correspondence to: ogonwosu2002@yahoo.com

References

[1] Jennette JC, Falk RJ. Glomerular clinicopathologic syndromes. In: Gilbert SJ, Weiner DE, editors. National Kidney Foundation's Primer on Kidney Diseases. 6th ed. Vol. 16. Philadelphia: Elsevier; 2014. pp. 162-163

[2] Madaio MP. Renal biopsy. Kidney International. 1990;**38**:529-543

[3] Iversen P, Brun C. Aspiration biopsy of the kidney. The American Journal of Medicine. 1951;**11**:324-330

[4] Korbet SM. Percutaneous renal biopsy. Seminars in Nephrology. 2002;**22**:254-267

[5] Maya ID, Maddela P, Barker J, Allon M. Percutaneous renal biopsy: Comparison of blind and real-time ultrasound-guided technique. Seminars in Dialysis. 2007;**20**:355-358

[6] Pasquariello A, Innocenti M, Batini V, Pasquariello G, Beati S, Rindi S, et al. Theoretical calculation of optimal depth in the percutaneous native kidney biopsy to drastically reduce bleeding complications and sample inadequacy for histopathological diagnosis. Nephrology, Dialysis, Transplantation. 2007;**22**:3516-3520

[7] Hogan JJ, Mocanu M, Berns JS. The native kidney biopsy: Update and evidence for best practice. Clinical Journal of the American Society of Nephrology. 2016;**11**:354-362

[8] Margaryan A, Perazella MA, Mahnensmith RL, Abu-Alfa AK. Experience with outpatient computed tomographic-guided renal biopsy. Clinical Nephrology. 2010;**74**:440-445

[9] Uppot RN, Harisinghani MG, Gervias DA. Imaging-guided percutaneous renal biopsy: Rationale and approach. AJR. 2010;**194**:1443-1449

[10] Mal F, Meyrier A, Callard P, Altman JJ, Kleinknecht D, Beaugrand M, et al. Transjugular renal biopsy. Lancet. 1990;**335**:1512-1513

[11] Rathod KR, Popat BA, Pandey A, Jamale TE, Hase NK, Deshmukh HL. Safety and effectiveness of transjugular renal biopsy: A single center study. Indian Journal of Nephrology. 2017;**27**:118-123. DOI: 10.4103/0971-4065.196932

[12] Gimenez LF, Micali S, Chen RN, Moore RG, Kavoussi LR, Scheel PJ Jr. Laparoscopic renal biopsy. Kidney International. 1998;**54**:525-529

[13] Shetye KR, Kavoussi LR, Ramakumar S, Fugita OE, Jarret TW. Laparoscopic renal biopsy: A 9-year experience. BJU International. 2003;**91**:817-820

[14] Walker PD, Cavallo T, Bonsib SM, The AdHoc Committee on Renal biopsy guidelines of the Renal Pathology Society. Practice guidelines for the renal biopsy. Modern Pathology. 2004;**17**:1555-1563

[15] Lee MW. Fusion imaging of real-time ultrasonography with CT or MRI for hepatic intervention. Ultrasonography. 2014;**33**:227-239

[16] Chung S, Koh ES, Kim SJ, Yoon HE, Park CW, Chang YS, et al. Safety and tissue yield for percutaneous native kidney biopsy according to practitioner and ultrasound technique. BMC Nephrology. 2014;**15**:96

[17] Burstein DM, Korbet SM, Schwartz MM. The use of the automatic core biopsy system in percutaneous renal biopsies: A comparative study. American Journal of Kidney Diseases. 1993;**22**:545-552

[18] Doyle AJ, Gregory MC, Terreros DA. Percutaneous native renal biopsy:

Comparison of a 1.2-mm spring-driven system with a traditional 2-mm hand-driven system. American Journal of Kidney Diseases. 1994;**23**:98-503

[19] Roth R, Parikh S, Makey D, Foster J, Rozenblit G, Satoskar A, et al. When size matters: Diagnostic value of kidney biopsy according to the gauge of the biopsy needle. American Journal of Nephrology. 2013;**37**:249-254

[20] Nicholson ML, Wheatley TJ, Doughman TM, White SA, Morgan JD, Veitch PS, et al. A prospective randomized trial of three different sizes of core-cutting needle for renal transplant biopsy. Kidney International. 2000;**58**:390-395

[21] Kriegshauser JS, Patel MD, Young SW, Chen F, Eversman WG, Chang YH, et al. Factors contributing to the success of ultrasound-guided native renal biopsy. Journal of Ultrasound in Medicine. 2016;**35**(2):381-387

[22] Pi X, Tang Z, Fu L, Guo M, Shi M, Chen L, et al. A new method of kidney biopsy using low dose CT-guidance with coaxial trocar and bard biopsy gun. BMC. 2013;**15**(1):1. DOI: 10.1186/1480-9222-15-1

[23] Mal F, Meyrier A, Callard P, Kleinknecht D, Altmann JJ, Beaugrand M. The diagnostic yield of transjugular renal biopsy. Experience in 200 cases. Kidney International. 1992;**41**:445-449

[24] Cluzel P, Martinez F, Bellin MF, Michalik Y, Beaufils H, Jouanneau C, et al. Transjugular versus percutaneous renal biopsy for the diagnosis of parenchymal disease: Comparison of sampling effectiveness and complications. Radiology. 2000;**215**:689-693

[25] Jouët P, Meyrier A, Mal F, Callard P, Guettier C, Stordeur D, et al. Transjugular renal biopsy in the treatment of patients with cirrhosis and renal abnormalities. Hepatology. 1996;**24**:1143-1147

[26] Rychlík I, Petrtýl J, Tesar V, Stejskalová A, Zabka J, Bruha R. Transjugular renal biopsy. Our experience with 67 cases. Kidney & Blood Pressure Research. 2001;**24**:207-212

[27] Thompson BC, Kingdon E, Johnston M, Tibballs J, Watkinson A, Jarmulowicz M, et al. Transjugular kidney biopsy. American Journal of Kidney Diseases. 2004;**43**:651-662

[28] Fine DM, Arepally A, Hofmann LV, Mankowitz SG, Atta MG. Diagnostic utility and safety of transjugular kidney biopsy in the obese patient. Nephrology, Dialysis, Transplantation. 2004;**19**:1798-1802

Chapter 4

Hemodialysis and Oral Health

Swati Jain, Kirti Jain and Basavaraj Patthi

Abstract

Changing lifestyle and sedentary schedule have led to the substantial increase in major noncommunicable diseases (NCDs) such as cardiac problems, cancers, diabetes, psychiatric disorders, and chronic respiratory diseases. Recent times have shown increased trends in incidence as well as prevalence of renal diseases. Hemodialysis is the most opted treatment modality for the patients of chronic renal diseases. Hence, the aim of the current chapter is to address the effect of renal diseases and its treatment on oral health. An extensive literature search from the year 2000 till 2015 was conducted to assess the effect of hemodialysis and renal diseases on various clinical parameters associated with oral health like dental caries, periodontal diseases, prevalence of calculus, etc. The literature review revealed that the dental health is compromised in the patients undergoing hemodialysis therapy. The oral health-related parameters get worsened with increasing duration of hemodialysis as well. The primary reason behind the debilitated periodontal condition among the patients may be attributed to the neglect of proper oral hygiene practices by the patient as they are preoccupied by more time-consuming and life-threatening kidney disease. A strong relation between oral health and hemodialysis has been observed. There is a need for further interdisciplinary research with emphasis on preventive dental treatment for the patients undergoing hemodialysis ensuring optimum outcome.

Keywords: hemodialysis, dental health, duration of dialysis, kidney diseases

1. Introduction

Healthy life is the most significant virtue of one's existence. The physical, social, and economical productivity of an individual depends mostly on the quality of life led by an individual. Human beings have always strived to achieve an optimum milieu of internal and external environment [1]. The diseases affecting mankind can be broadly classified into two types—communicable and noncommunicable diseases. With improvement in health-care facilities, sanitation, litigation services, and treatment modalities, the reign of communicable diseases is on a decline. However, a contrary rise of noncommunicable diseases (NCDs) has been observed primarily due to changing lifestyles and diet [2].

The changing scenario favoring NCDs can primarily be contributed to sedentary lifestyle and rapid population aging especially in developing countries like India. Diseases like cardiac problems, cancers, diabetes, psychiatric disorders, and chronic respiratory diseases have seen an exponential increase in recent times and have become the leading causes of death globally killing more people each year than all other causes combined [2, 3]. As per the Global Burden of Disease Study for 1990, noncommunicable diseases ranked first as the cause of death in developed countries as well as in many developing countries and the world as a whole. Hence, common risk factor approach addressing the problems and issues connected with noncommunicable diseases can influence the major health gains worldwide [3, 4].

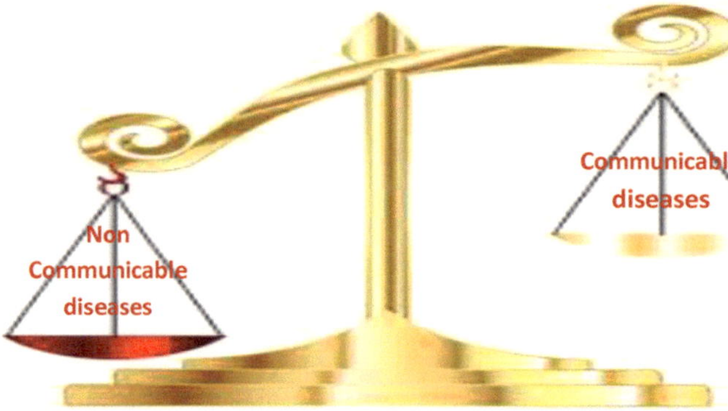

CHANGING PARADIM OF DISEASES

2. Kidney diseases

Kidneys play one of the vital roles in human beings as excretory organs. Their major functions include excretion of metabolic wastes, electrolyte regulation, and endocrine regulatory functions. Each human kidney is composed of about one million anatomical and functional units called nephron which is further composed of glomerule and tubule. Renal diseases pose a major health problem of modern world [5]. Compromised renal function might lead finally to renal failure which is characterized by the loss of functional capacity of nephrons associated with reduced glomerular functional rate [6]. The most frequent etiology of chronic renal failure includes diabetes mellitus, hypertension, glomerulonephritis, polycystic kidney disease, and pyelonephritis. Previously, glomerulonephritis was known to be the main cause of chronic renal failure; however, now diabetes mellitus and hypertension are the etiologic factors of the disease today which are considered to have genetic origin mostly [7, 8].

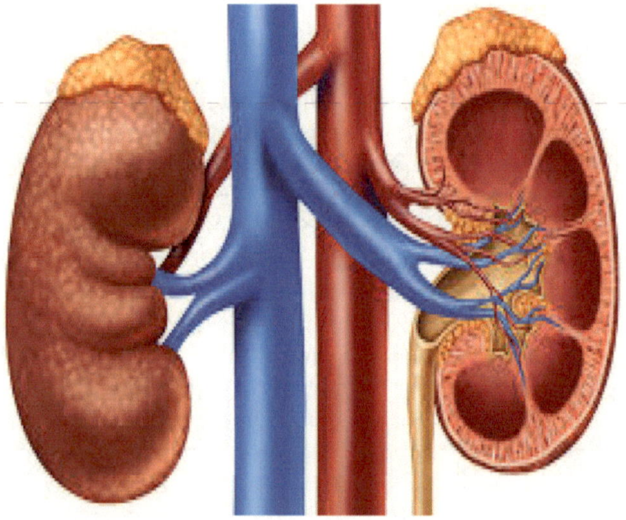

Transplantation is the ideal treatment for patients with end-stage renal disease. But, due to limited availability of matched donors for kidney transplantation, there has been an increased focus on alternative treatment modalities like hemodialysis and peritoneal dialysis. In the last three to four decades, improvements in dialysis and transplantation have reduced morbidity and mortality among patients with end-stage renal disease.

3. Hemodialysis and oral health

Hemodialysis treatment modality is usually prescribed for prolonged duration with weekly frequency of once, twice, or more than twice a week, thus, creating a stressful environment for the patients [9]. This long-standing treatment modality has affected the survival rate among the patients positively. However, the chronic condition might influence the incidence of other systemic diseases in these patients primarily due to the lack of their ability to control water and electrolyte balance and filtrate waste products [10].

Further, oral health among these patients undergoing hemodialysis has been reported to be poor primarily due to their delicate state, neglect of oral hygiene, manifestations of systemic conditions, and immunosuppression [11, 12]. The specific effects of chronic renal disease and renal replacement therapy on periodontal tissues include gingival hyperplasia, increased level of plaque, calculus, and destructive periodontal disease. The findings have been reported by many studies [10, 13, 14]. It is interesting to note further that the dental diseases have coherent relation with the treatment duration of hemodialysis as well [8]. Very few studies have presented a cumulative data concerning the effect of duration of hemodialysis therapy on oral health of the patients undergoing hemodialysis. Hence the present chapter gives an insight of the oral health manifestations of hemodialysis and the underlying kidney disease correlating it with the duration of the treatment modality.

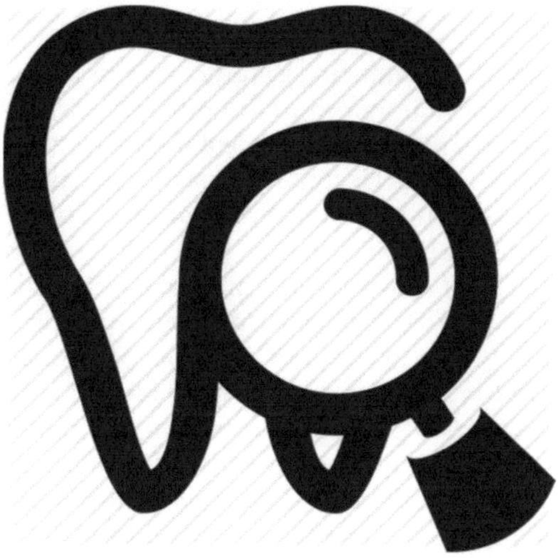

4. Influence of hemodialysis on oral health according to various studies

Hemodialysis has emerged as an optimum treatment modality for the patients with compromised renal function significantly reducing the mortality rate of these diseases. Researchers have provided with substantial evidence that chronic systemic diseases like renal failure and its treatment modalities have a significant effect on the oral environment resulting in an increased burden of oral diseases among these

S. No.	Oral findings in hemodialysis patients	Previous studies
1.	Debilitated periodontal status	1. Klassen and Krasko [7] 2. Bayraktar et al. [16] 3. Torkzaban et al. [10] 4. Joseph [13] 5. Dencheva [17] 6. Malekmakan [12] 7. Parkar et al. [11] 8. Bhatsange et al. [19] 9. Ziebolz et al. [20] 10. Jenabian et al. [8] 11. Kaushik et al. [21] 12. Jain et al. [23]
2.	Poor dental caries status	1. Dumitrescu et al. [18] 2. Ziebolz et al. [20]
3.	Poor oral hygiene behavior	1. Klassen and Krasko [7] 2. Dumitrescu et al. [18] 3. Xie et al. [22]
4.	Neglected oral health care seeking behavior among hemodialysis patients	1. Klassen and Krasko [7] 2. Dumitrescu et al. [18] 3. Xie et al. [22] 4. Jain et al. [23]
5.	Increased salivary buffer capacity	1. Ertugrul [14] 2. Kaushik et al. [21]

Table 1.
Oral health and hemodialysis: summary of literature review.

patients [2, 10, 11]. An insight into the various studies conducted worldwide would help us understand the topic (**Table 1**).

1. **Klassen and Krasko** [7] conducted a study to assess the dental health of dialysis patients. A questionnaire and a noninvasive oral examination were obtained from hemodialysis and peritoneal dialysis patients registered in the dialysis program at St. Paul's Hospital in Saskatoon, Saskatchewan. A detailed medical history was obtained and recorded of a total of 373 dialysis patients in Central and Northern Saskatchewan. The clinical examination revealed that 64% of the patients who were dentate had been on dialysis for a mean of more than 2 years. Majority of the patients were diabetic, and almost all were hypertensive. Sixty (64%) of the dentate patients were candidates for kidney transplantation. The oral findings revealed an increased prevalence of tooth mobility, fractures, erosion, attrition, recession, gingivitis, and a high plaque index. Majority of the patients reported brushing once or more daily, but they flossed infrequently or never. Dental visits were infrequent, less than every 5 years in 59 (63%) of the dentate patients. Almost 81% of the treating dentists were aware about the medical condition of their patients. The author has concluded that the oral health of hemodialysis patients was compromised and required urgent attention and intervention.

2. **Ertugrul** [14] assessed the oral health status of children suffering from end-stage renal disease identifying the causes of low caries prevalence in this population in comparison with the control group. The study group consisted of 38 children, aged 4–17 years being treated in pediatric nephrology units at three different hospitals in Izmir, Turkey. The study and control groups had similar baseline oral hygiene habits with respect to daily tooth brushing

frequency and periodic dental checkup frequency. Oral examination findings indicated severe enamel hypoplasia in the study group with significant difference for DMFT and gingival and plaque indices when compared with the control group. It was further observed that study group showed high salivary buffer capacity in 89.5% of patients. Salivary levels of cariogenic streptococcus mutans and lactobacilli in the study group were significantly lower than in the control group. It was concluded that high salivary buffer capacity was observed due to increased concentrations of antibacterial chemicals such as urea in the saliva of children with ESRD. Also decreased levels of cariogenic microorganisms were detected. Thus, the authors suggested that all hemodialysis patients should receive dental health education, including oral hygiene instruction, in order to improve their overall oral health.

3. **Marakogolu et al.** [15] **carried out a study** to assess the microbial dental plaque load among the patients undergoing hemodialysis. For clinical parameters, gingival Index (GI), plaque index (PI) scores, and probing depths (PD) were recorded for hemodialysis patients and controls matched with the patient group. However, the results showed no statistically significant difference regarding clinical parameters between the two groups attributed mostly to the small sample size evaluated.

4. **Bayraktar et al.** [16] compared the periodontal and oral health status of hemodialysis patients and healthy controls. Seventy-six hemodialysis patients and 61 controls were examined for plaque deposits, gingivitis, periodontitis, calculus accumulation, and oral health status. The results showed no statistical difference in the probing pocket depths (PPD) but a highly significant difference for plaque index ($P < 0.001$), gingival index (GI) ($P = 0.007$), and calculus surface index ($P < 0.001$). There was a highly significant difference for GI ($P = 0.001$) and PPD scores ($P < 0.001$) between subgroups receiving hemodialysis 3 years or more. A positive correlation between time on dialysis and parameter of missing teeth, GI scores, and measurement of PPD was found in the patient group. The hemodialysis group showed less DMFT than the controls.

5. **Torkzaban et al.** [10] conducted a survey to assess the prevalence of periodontal disease and its related characteristics in 31 hemodialysis patients from the dialysis department of educational Ekbatan Hospital in Hamadan. Clinical parameters that were assessed were periodontal disease index (PDI), papillary bleeding index (PBI), and plaque control record index (PCRI), and medical history was recorded. Then, the recorded data were analyzed. It was observed that all hemodialysis patients had periodontal disease. Plaque control record index was higher than 50% in nearly all patients. Despite the high accumulation of plaque in the patients, the rate of gingival bleeding was low. Also, it was observed that more than half of the patients did not brush their teeth. Renal transplantation patients had a lower plaque accumulation than the others, and consequently periodontal disease was less observed. Periodontal condition debilitated with the duration of hemodialysis.

6. **Joseph** [13] carried out a study with an aim to assess the prevalence of periodontal disease among a group of patients with renal disease and healthy controls. A total of 77 renal disease patients and 77 healthy controls were examined for clinical parameters like oral hygiene status, gingival inflammation, probing pocket depth, and clinical attachment loss. Periodontal findings

were grouped into three as no/mild, moderate, and severe periodontitis. All periodontal parameters were significantly high in patients as compared to controls ($p < 0.001$). The prevalence and severity of periodontal disease was also significantly higher in the case group ($p < 0.001$). This study provides evidence for a greater prevalence and severity of periodontal disease among patients with renal disease. The periodontal health of all patients with renal disease needs to be carefully monitored.

7. **Dencheva** [17] conducted a study to estimate the periodontal conditions and treatment needs by CPITN of 150 patients out of which 45 (30%) were on hemodialysis, 45 (30%) were renal transplanted patients, and 60 (40%) were healthy controls, aged between 18 and 84 years. All patients were asked not to brush their teeth before the examination. Periodontal examination was done after dialysis. The results showed that CPI score 3 and CPI score 2 in the control group were more significant than those in hemodialysis groups and transplanted group. Sixty percent from transplanted group have gingival pockets of up to 3.5 mm and sub- and/or supragingival calculus. The percentage of patients with code CPI 3 is also high and shallow. Most patients in control group (71%) were with CPI 2. None of the three groups of patients with healthy periodontium in all sextants existed.

8. **Dumitrescu et al.** [18] assessed oral health status and behaviors among Romanian adult individuals on renal dialysis along with self-reported anxiety, stress, and depression level. A cross-sectional study was conducted on a total sample size of 61 adults (mean age 53.9 years; 44% women; 66% married). The questionnaire included information about sociodemographic factors, behavioral factors, self-reported oral health status, anxiety, stress, and depression. The clinical parameters revealed that 99.4% of the participants reported to have current non-treated caries, 94.4% were not satisfied by appearance of own teeth, 97.5% presented extracted teeth, and 64.6% of them reported to have gum bleeding. 34.5% of the individuals brushed once a day or less, 92.5% of them never used dental floss, and 78.3% never used mouth rinse. Regarding oral hygiene practices, only 13% of participants availed dental treatment services, and 89.4% had consulted the dentist only when treatment is needed or when in pain. The main reasons for non-consultation from a dentist were anxiety and financial roadblock. A high percentage of dialysis patients presented anxiety (85.1%), stress (60.9%), and depression in everyday life (61.5%). Duration of hemodialysis did not affect the clinical oral parameters examined. The results supported the view that there was an increased risk for anxiety, stress, depression, and impaired dental/gingival health and behaviors among individuals on renal dialysis. Early dental treatment and psychological interventions were recommended.

9. **Malekmakan** [12] aimed to assess the oral health status and related risk factors in Iranian hemodialysis patients. Sociodemographic information, medical history, and dental health findings were recorded for 72 patients (mean age and HD time of 53.4 ± 15.3 years and 36.9 ± 33.8 months, respectively). The results showed that 48.6% of the patients complained of dry mouth, 49.3% of taste change, and 31% of bad breath. A high 46.9% of the hemodialysis patients had dental calculus. The mean DMFT score was 18.6 ± 9.9. The authors observed that DMFT score was significantly lower in patients with dental calculus than in patients without it ($P = 0.001$).

10. **Parkar et al.** [11] assessed the periodontal status of patients in hemodialysis patients in two super specialty renal institutes in Gujarat, India, through a cross-sectional study in 152 hemodialysis patients and 152 controls. Clinical parameters were evaluated through simplified oral hygiene index, community periodontal index (CPI), and loss of attachment (LOA) as per WHO methodology 1997. The findings of the study highlighted that the dialysis group had compromised oral hygiene than controls (**P** < 0.001). There was a high severity of periodontitis in the dialysis group as compared with the control group (**P** < 0.001). None of the subjects had healthy periodontium. There was a high severity of periodontitis (for both in terms of CPI and LOA) in the dialysis group as compared with control group that was found to be statistically highly significant (**P** < 0.001). For the intergroup comparison for CPI and LOA, there was no statistical significant difference regarding the periodontal findings. It was thus concluded that periodontal diseases are prevalent in chronic renal failure patients emphasizing the need for concurrent dental treatment among these patients.

11. **Bhatsange et al.** [19] conducted a study to gain an insight into whether duration of dialysis therapy influences the oral and periodontal health of hemodialysis patients. A total of 75 hemodialysis patients and 25 controls was assessed. Depending upon the duration of dialysis, the study groups were divided into three subgroups. Simplified oral hygiene index and periodontal disease index by Ramfjord were recorded. The results showed that the prevalence of periodontal disease was evident in the dialysis group. Oral hygiene status was poor in comparison with the control group. Clinical and biochemical parameters showed a statistically significant difference between the groups rather than within the groups.

12. **Ziebolz et al.** [20] evaluated oral hygiene behavior and oral health status of hemodialysis patients in Germany. Dental examination findings consisted of DMFT and the degree of gingival inflammation (PDI: periodontal disease index) among 129 patients. The findings revealed the average dialysis duration was 4.1 years. The underlying kidney diseases were glomerulonephritis in 30% of patients and diabetic nephropathy in 22% of patients. Only 63% of the patients (n = 34) visited a dentist when they had complaints. In 46 cases (85%), the dentist had been informed about the patient's requirement for dialysis, and in most cases (70%), the dental treatment took place on the day after dialysis. The clinical parameters showed that the mean DMFT of the patients was 22.1 ± 6.5. The median degree of gingival inflammation (PDI) was 1. In addition to a high proportion of missing teeth, a good level of restoration of caries was found. The gingiva showed only a low level of inflammatory changes.

13. **Jenabian et al.** [8] assessed the periodontal status of hemodialysis patients in Babol, Northern Iran. A total of 115 patients were studied (63 males, 52 females). The clinical parameters which were assessed were plaque index (PI), gingival index (GI), clinical attachment level (CAL), and probing pocket depth (PPD). The data were collected and analyzed. The results showed that PI, GI, CAL, and PPD scores were 2.37 ± 0.55, 2.36 ± 0.63, 3.98 ± 1.61, and 4.41 ± 1.4, respectively. It was observed that the PI scores deteriorated with increasing age (p < 0.024). Also, CAL was significantly higher in males than in females (4.39 ± 1.57 vs. 3.53 ± 1.56, p < 0.02). The results showed that longer duration of hemodialysis is associated with severe periodontal diseases, especially in males.

14. **Kaushik et al.** [21] assessed the changing oral and salivary environment in patients suffering from end-stage renal disease (ESRD) and undergoing hemodialysis. A cross-sectional study was conducted on 100 ESRD patients over a period of 15 months out of which 25 patients were randomly selected to assess the salivary changes and compared with 25 controls. The study showed that most common oral manifestations in these patients were oral malodor, dry mouth, taste change, increased caries incidence, calculus formation, and gingival bleeding. The salivary findings revealed that the rates of both unstimulated and stimulated whole saliva decreased in patients; however, pH and buffer capacity of unstimulated whole saliva increased. The authors have suggested that ESRD patients undergoing hemodialysis require special considerations during dental treatment as they have varied oral manifestations primarily due to their treatment modality.

15. **Xie et al.** [22] evaluated oral health status and oral hygiene behavior among hemodialysis patients in China. Caries status was examined and recorded along with the sociodemographic information of 306 patients, aged 24–88 (58.09 ± 14.06). It was interesting to note that that majority of the patients followed good oral hygiene practices and brushed their teeth twice daily. However, limited use of other oral hygiene aids like floss or mouth wash was reported. The oral health treatment seeking behavior was compromised since the commencement of hemodialysis therapy. The mean DMFT scores of the patient were 9.63 ± 7.54. It was concluded that hemodialysis therapy seemed to prevent patients from visiting a dentist and there was a great need for dental treatment among these patients.

16. **Jain et al.** [23] conducted a study to assess the effect of duration of hemodialysis and the underlying kidney disease on the dental health status of patients undergoing hemodialysis and to compare their dental health status with that of healthy controls. A cross-sectional study was conducted on 400 patients and 400 controls selected through stratified random sampling method from five zones of Delhi. Based on the duration of hemodialysis, the patient group was divided into subgroups ranging from less than 3 months to more than 12 months. The complete oral health status was recorded using the WHO dentition status and treatment need, community periodontal index, oral hygiene index, and prosthetic status and prosthetic needs. It was observed that with increasing duration of hemodialysis, periodontal status worsened as per maximum CPI scores (p value = 0.018). Majority of patients (81.25%) reported the presence of calculus. It was interesting to observe that the severity of periodontal disease was higher among the patient group (p value 0.035). Oral hygiene status was also compromised among patients (mean OHI scores 5.15 ± 1.975). No significant difference was observed regarding caries status among patients and controls. Prosthetic needs were higher among patients. It was thus concluded that the duration of hemodialysis had a significant influence on oral hygiene status and prosthetic needs signifying the need of preventive dental treatment.

5. Discussion and summary

The present chapter highlights the fact that oral health status is debilitated and compromised among the hemodialysis patients and gets worsened with increasing duration and hemodialysis and underlying kidney disease which might contribute significantly to morbidity and potential mortality among these patients. This further emphasizes the concept of common risk factor approach with multidisciplinary patient care approach.

The dental health is compromised in patients undergoing hemodialysis therapy, and with the increasing duration of hemodialysis, various clinical oral health-related parameters get worsened with increasing duration of hemodialysis. The chronic disease condition and time-taking treatment (hemodialysis) affect the oral health-care habits resulting in poor periodontal condition among the patients. The psychological effect of long-standing kidney diseases resulting in high stress level and depression in hemodialysis patients compromises the periodontal health further. Hence, oral health promotive and preventive intervention early in the hemodialysis patients can influence the oral health status positively.

This warrants the need for intensified preventive oral health-care modalities in these patients, so as to improve their dental health which can have a significant impact on their overall health. The dialysis team should be encouraged to make the dental referral as early as possible, if needed, and regular monthly dental checkups should be advocated. Further emphasis on the effective implementation of oral health promotion program for medically compromised patients is recommended. Oral health education and counseling regarding oral health-care-seeking behavior during the hemodialysis appointment can motivate and educate patients along with their family members. At the same time, dental fraternity should receive appropriate training for treatment of these medically compromised patients to cater to the needs of this special group.

Analysis of the effect of duration of dialysis on the periodontal tissues did not show confirmatory relationship. However the frequency of hemodialysis has a significant influence on the periodontal status of the patients with a deteriorated CPI scores with the increased frequency of hemodialysis from once to twice and more than twice a week.

Also, there is a significant existence of higher prosthetic needs concerning to mouth among the patients undergoing hemodialysis. Hence, oral health-care delivery system may be strengthened to cater to the prosthetic needs of these patients as well. Increased prosthetic needs of the patients with the duration of dialysis might be attributed to the dental care denial by the dental practitioners owing to their compromised medical status.

The hemodialysis patients usually report poor oral hygiene. These patients exhibit immunocompromised state although they are not completely immune deficient and are still able to deal with bacterial challenge. The patients with chronic kidney disease showed poor oral hygiene which could probably be due to long-standing disease duration leading to a debilitated oral hygiene. Further there is high deposit of calculus on teeth due to uremic salivary pH in hemodialysis patients.

Majority of the hemodialysis patients suffer from diabetic nephropathy and have strict dietary pattern. Further, increased alkalinity of the oral cavity is reported in the uremic patients as a result of high urea level in saliva inhibiting bacterial growth and increasing salivary buffer capacity [23].

Further studies are required to correlate the dental findings with the biochemical serum markers over a duration of time so as to validate the influence of duration of dialysis therapy on dental health.

The current chapter highlights the relation between oral health and hemodialysis. This further necessitates more interdisciplinary research on this topic. Medical and dental health-care professionals need to join hands and work together ensuring optimum patient care.

Author details

Swati Jain[1*], Kirti Jain[2] and Basavaraj Patthi[3]

1 National Health Mission, Maulana Azad Institute of Dental Sciences, New Delhi, India

2 Ashok Multispeciality Hospital, New Delhi, India

3 Department of Public Health Dentistry, Divya Jyoti College of Dental Sciences and Research, India

*Address all correspondence to: doc_bk2@yahoo.co.in

References

[1] World Health Organization. Ottawa Charter for Health Promotion. Europe; 1986. pp. 1-5

[2] World Health Organization. Global Status Report on Non Communicable Diseases. Italy: WHO Press; 2010. pp. 1-11

[3] FDI. FDI Policy Statement-Non-Communicable Diseases. Hong Kong: FDI General Assembly; 2012. pp. 1-3

[4] Nissinen A, Berios X, Puska P. Community based non communicable disease interventions: Lessons from developed countries for developing ones. Bulletin of the World Health Organization. 2001;**79**(10):963-970

[5] Cervero AJ, Bagan JV, Soriano YJ, Roda RP. Dental management in renal failure: Patients on Dialysis. Medicina Oral, Patología Oral y Cirugía Bucal. 2008;**13**(7):E419-E426

[6] Zhang QL, Rothenbacher D. Prevalence of chronic kidney disease in population-based studies: Systematic review. BMC Public Health. 2008;**8**:11-40

[7] Klassen JT, Krasko BM. The dental health status of dialysis patients. Journal of the Canadian Dental Association. 2002;**68**(1):34-38

[8] Jenabian N, Mirsaeed AMG, Ehsani H, Kiakojori A. Periodontal status of patient' underwent hemodialysis therapy. Caspian Journal of Internal Medicine. 2013;**4**(2):658-661

[9] Sullivan JD. End stage renal disease economics and the balance of treatment modalities. Journal of Service Science & Management. 2010;**3**:45-50

[10] Torkzaban P, Arabi R, Kadkhodazadeh M, Moradi J, Khoshhal M. Periodontal status in patients undergoing hemodialysis. Dental Journal of Hamadan University of Medical Sciences. 2009;**1**(1):7-10

[11] Parkar SM, Ajithkrishnan CG. Periodontal status in patients undergoing hemodialysis. Indian Journal of Nephrology. 2012;**22**(4):246-250

[12] Malekmakan L, Haghpanah S, Pakfetrat M, Ebrahimic Z, Hasanlic E. Oral health status in Iranian hemodialysis patients. Indian Journal of Nephrology. 2011;**21**(4):235-238

[13] Joseph R, Krishnan R, Narayan V. Higher prevalence of periodontal disease among patients with predialytic renal disease. Brazilian Journal of Oral Sciences. 2009;**8**(1):14-18

[14] Ertugrul F, Elbek-Cubukçu C, Sabah E, Mir S. The oral health status of children undergoing hemodialysis treatment. The Turkish Journal of Pediatrics. 2003;**45**(2):108-113

[15] Marakogolu I, Gursoy UK, Demirer S, Sezer H. Periodontal patients of chronic renal failure patients receiving hemodialysis. Yonsei Medical Journal. 2003;**44**(4):648-652

[16] Bayraktar G et al. Dental and periodontal findings in hemodialysis patients. Oral Diseases. 2007;**13**(4):393-397

[17] Dencheva M. Research of periodontal status and treatment needs by CPITN in patients on haemodialysis and renal transplanted patients. Journal of IMAB – Annual Proceeding (Scientific Papers). 2009;**2**:1-3

[18] Dumitrescu AL, Garnieta L, Guzun O. Anxiety, stress, depression, oral health status and behaviours in Romanian hemodialysis patients. Romanian Journal of Internal Medicine. 2009;**47**(2):161-168

[19] Bhatsange A, Patil SR. Assessment of periodontal health status in patients undergoing renal dialysis: A descriptive, cross-sectional study. Journal of Indian Society of Periodontology. 2012 Jan;**16**(1):37-42

[20] Ziebolz D, Fischer P, Hornecker E, Mausberg RE. Oral health of hemodialysis patients: A cross-sectional study at two German dialysis centers. Hemodialysis International. 2012;**16**(1):69-75

[21] Kaushik A, Reddy SS, Umesh L, Devi B, Santana N, Rakesh N. Oral and salivary changes among renal patients undergoing hemodialysis: A cross sectional study. Indian Journal of Nephrology. 2013;**23**:123-129

[22] Xie T, Yang Z, Dai G, Yan K, Tian Y, Zhao D, et al. Evaluation of the oral health status in Chinese hemodialysis patients. Hemodialysis International. 2014;**18**(3):668-673

[23] Jain S, Singla A, Basavaraj P, Singh S, Singh K, Kundu H. Underlying kidney disease and duration of hemodialysis: An assessment of its effect on oral health. Journal of Clinical and Diagnostic Research. 2014;**8**(5):ZC65-ZC69

Chapter 5

Post-Biopsy Complications Associated with Percutaneous Kidney Biopsy

Paulo Ramos Botelho Antunes, Stanley Almeida Araújo, Silvana Maria Carvalho Miranda, Fabiano Franco Monteiro Prado, Luiz Felipe França Antunes, Elisa Carvalho de Siqueira, Fabrício Tinôco Alvim de Souza and Maria Carolina Barbosa Álvares

Abstract

Renal physiology and physiopathology have been the object of studies aimed at developing exams that can assist in the early diagnosis of the base disease. Chronic kidney disease consists of the progressive, irreversible loss of kidney function. Early detection and appropriate treatment can minimize the progression of the disease, lower the inherent costs, and improve the quality of life of affected individuals. Kidney biopsy is the key method in this evaluation, as it enables the histological and immunohistochemical analysis of specimens in a fast, safe, and economical manner. The main indications for kidney biopsy are nephrotic syndrome, acute kidney failure of unknown etiology, persistent hematuria and proteinuria, chronic kidney disease with conserved kidney dimensions, and transplanted kidneys (to evaluate stages of rejection, infection, and/or sclerosis). However, as an invasive method, kidney biopsy is not without complications. Post-biopsy complication rates range from 5 to 15%, with 6.6% considered minor (macrohematuria with no need for blood transfusion) and another 7.7% considered major (hemorrhage requiring blood transfusion or other approaches). In this chapter, we address the main aspects of kidney biopsy, the technical procedures for its execution, and the management of the main complications stemming from this procedure.

Keywords: kidney biopsy, percutaneous kidney biopsy, post-biopsy complications, complications, ultrasound-guided biopsy

1. Introduction

Renal lesions are subdivided based on duration as acute kidney injury (AKI) and chronic kidney disease (CKD). AKI has numerous hemodynamic, inflammatory, toxic, and obstructive causes, which, when diagnosed and treated early, can be reversed, thereby avoiding permanent damage [1, 2]. CKD, however, is the clinical detection of a progressive, irreversible loss of kidney function, for which the aim of therapy is to minimize the progression of the disease [2].

Percutaneous kidney biopsy has become part of clinical practice in nephrology, as it enables the diagnosis, prognostic assessment, and therapeutic guidance of kidney diseases [3, 4]. Since its advent in the 1950s, advances have been achieved in the technique to improve the diagnostic yield and minimize complications [5].

2. Percutaneous ultrasound-guided renal biopsy

2.1 Indications

The indication for a kidney biopsy is determined mainly by signs and symptoms [4]. The global rate of biopsy (number of procedures per million [ppm]) in native kidneys ranges from more than 250 ppm in Australia to less than 75 ppm in the United States. This divergence in kidney biopsy rates is influenced by the prevalence of kidney disease as well as different opinions regarding the value of the procedure in terms of diagnosis, prognosis, and therapy [6].

The main objectives that lead to the indication for kidney biopsy are the need for a precise diagnosis and treatment, the need to determine the degree of activity and chronicity of the lesion in order to establish the prognosis and possible response to treatment, and the evaluation of genetic diseases [6]. The diagnostic contribution of a kidney biopsy is undeniable in cases of nephrotic syndrome, systemic disease kidney failure, unexplained AKI, and transplanted kidney dysfunction [7].

For cases of idiopathic nephrotic syndrome in adults and children older than 6 years of age, the indication for a kidney biopsy is extremely important, as the findings often influence therapeutic decision-making [8]. In a prospective study involving 276 biopsies of native kidneys, the diagnosis resulting from the biopsy influenced the management of 86% of cases of nephrotic syndrome [9]. However, there is a variety of clinical situations of nephrotic syndrome for which a kidney biopsy is not generally performed at the time of diagnosis, such as in cases of children between 1 and 6 years of age due to the high prevalence of minimal change disease [10, 11]. In such situations, corticotherapy is indicated and biopsy is only performed in cases of therapeutic failure or the appearance of another sign or symptom not associated with minimal change disease [11]. Biopsy is also not performed initially in cases of secondary nephrotic disease clearly associated with the introduction of a medication known to cause this condition, such as non-steroidal anti-inflammatory drugs, gold salts, pamidronate, penicillamine, and lithium. This group includes patients with longstanding diabetes with gradual proteinuria progression, those with morbid obesity and slowly increasing proteinuria accompanied or not by diabetes and worsening kidney function, those with systemic diseases such as primary or secondary amyloidosis in which the diagnosis can be made through less invasive methods, such as adipose tissue biopsy, and patients known to have malignant diseases involving nephrotic syndrome [6]. Patients with nephrotic syndrome generally exhibit hematuria, proteinuria, hypertension, and renal dysfunction, and the condition is also often associated with systemic diseases. Therefore, kidney biopsy contributes to the diagnosis, therapeutic decision-making, and classification of the disease (e.g., systemic lupus erythematosus). In suspected cases of post-streptococcal glomerulonephritis, biopsy is only recommended when a gradual worsening in serum levels of creatinine, prolonged hypocomplementemia, and recurring hematuria are observed [6, 7].

Cases of systemic diseases with kidney failure include non-nephrotic proteinuria, isolated glomerular hematuria, and unexplained CKD. Protein is a marker and factor related to the progression of kidney disease. Studies have demonstrated a relation between the degree of proteinuria and the progression of CKD in cases of non-nephrotic proteinuria [7]. Thus, many nephrologists routinely perform a kidney biopsy in patients with higher non-nephrotic proteinuria (1–2 g/day) in the absence of another clinical condition that might explain the findings (e.g., diabetes mellitus or hypertension). However, in situations of low-grade proteinuria (500–1000 mg/day) in the absence of glomerular hematuria, altered kidney function, and clinical/serological evidence of a systemic disease, a biopsy is generally not performed [6]. Biopsy in cases of isolated glomerular hematuria remains controversial, as the procedure exerts little influence on therapeutic decision-making. When performed, the conditions most often encountered are Alport syndrome, thin basement membrane nephropathy, and immunoglobulin A nephropathy. In a prospective analysis, biopsy influenced the therapeutic decision-making in only one of the 36 procedures performed [9]. For patients with unexplained CKD, a kidney biopsy can provide important information, despite the greater risk of complication. In cases of exacerbated CKD, a biopsy may reveal lesions that can be treated and reversed. Moreover, a biopsy can contribute important knowledge to clinical management in cases of the need for a kidney transplant [7].

For patients with unexplained AKI, biopsy is indicated in cases of an uncertain etiology and can influence clinical management in 71% of cases [9]. Biopsy is also particularly useful for early or late-onset dysfunction of a renal graft. In cases of acute graft dysfunction, the procedure enables confirming the diagnosis of rejection and specifying the pathological mechanism (acute cellular rejection or antibody mediated rejection). Late biopsies also furnish essential information to assist in differentiating the causes of chronic nephropathy of the graft, such as chronic rejection, transplant glomerulopathy, nephrotoxicity, viral disease, lymphoproliferative diseases, and relapse of the base disease. The simplicity of the technical procedure and richness of the diagnostic and prognostic information make biopsy indispensable to the follow-up of renal grafts [7].

Contraindications for kidney biopsy may be absolute or relative. For percutaneous kidney biopsies, absolute contraindications include uncontrolled severe hypertension, the inability of the patient to cooperate with the biopsy, having only one kidney, and uncontrollable hemorrhagic diathesis, whereas relative contraindications include severe azotemia, anatomic kidney abnormalities, anticoagulation, pregnancy, and urinary tract infection [3].

2.2 Techniques and materials

Kidney biopsies can be guided by different imaging methods, the most common of which are ultrasound (US) and computed tomography (CT) due to their good performance and broad availability. In contrast, magnetic resonance is employed little due to the greater cost and need for specific material. The choice between US and CT should be individualized and based on the physician's experience, kidney volume, location of the biopsy site, patient's clinical condition, and the availability of the equipment. US is generally the imaging method of choice for guiding a kidney biopsy, since it enables obtaining samples from virtually any site and visualizing the needle in real time. It also does not expose the patient to radiation, can be performed in any environment, including at the bedside, and enables the continual monitoring of any pre-operative complications. It is also the method of choice for post-procedure follow-up, enabling the early detection of complications [4].

To be successful, US-guided kidney biopsy requires specific conditions. The patient must be placed in ventral decubitus on the examining table and the procedure must be performed in a sterile environment. The transducer should be covered with a sterile film. There are specific transducer covers on the market, but a sterile glove can be used in cases of emergency. Antisepsis should be performed on the entire side of the back corresponding to the kidney to be biopsied. The selection of the puncture site is determined by US considering the best path (least distance between the skin and renal capsule and the absence of vascular structures and/or interposed intestinal loops). This region in the center of the US image ensures the safest path for the biopsy and provides better control and resolution of the image.

Once the region to be punctured has been defined, the skin at the puncture site is anesthetized and the area of anesthesia is then extended to the deep layers, preferably reaching the perirenal layers, including adjacencies external to Gerota's fascia and the renal capsule. An alternative is the use of a long 18G peripheral intravenous catheter with the administration of 20 ml of anesthetic solution (10 ml of 2% xylocaine with no vasoconstrictor +10 ml of 0.9% saline solution or bi-distilled water). The entire anesthetic procedure as well as the subsequent steps should be guided by US. Some authors prefer performing a biopsy with their hands free. The two techniques (with or without US) have the same rates of minor and major complications and obtain adequate material for analysis, but the hands-free method requires greater experience and has a somewhat slower learning curve [1, 12]. Next, the biopsy needle is aligned with the transducer (when US is used) and introduced at a 45° angle to the skin. To ensure the safety of the procedure and control of complications, both the needle and its path should be kept within the US viewing field. The path to follow with the needle in the renal parenchyma should only involve the renal cortex (glomerular region), without transfixing the renal medulla, which contributes little to the study and has large-caliber vessels that could be associated with vascular complications; this also avoids the occurrence of injury to the renal calyces and pelvis [4, 13]. The number of fragments to collect depends on the number and types of exams requested as well as the presence of the pathologist during the exam, who may express opinions regarding the quality of the specimen collected. In procedures without the presence of a pathologist, two fragments are normally collected for each exam solicited.

Different needle calibers, lengths, and tip shapes are available on the market for the collection of material for microscopic analysis. Thin-needle punctures are performed with calibers ranging from 20 to 25, whereas thick-needle biopsies are performed with 14- to 19-gauge needles. Authors state that thin needles provide smaller fragments for analysis, but the fragments have similar quality and anatomopathological interpretation to those obtained with thick needles. Nonetheless, larger fragments enable a more complete study of renal pathologies. Moreover, although a smaller caliber is related to a lower rate of complications stemming from the procedure, it does not assist in the renal evaluation [14]. Along with a core biopsy needle (thick needle), coaxial needles can be used, which have a larger diameter with sufficient inner diameter to enable the navigation of the core biopsy needle in its interior. The use of coaxial needle kits avoids multiple punctures of the capsule, as this mechanism enables acquiring several tissue samples with a single perforation, which reduces the procedure time. However, portions of the organ cannot be sampled with this method and the use of such needles increases the cost of the procedure. The use of coaxial needles enables the operator to easily embolize the needle path with an absorbable gelatin sponge when removing the outer needle at the end of the procedure. This embolization promoted by the coaxial method is believed to reduce the risks of post-biopsy bleeding, but this characteristic is reported to not be an advantage of the method. Thus, both the coaxial and non-coaxial techniques do not appear to influence the bleeding complication rate [15]. The use of spring-loaded tools is currently recommended. These needles are classified based on the form of discharge into the tissue: automatic or semi-automatic (disposable). Such tools are reported to be more effective and safer than classic percutaneous renal biopsies that use the Tru-Cut or Vim-Silverman needle. Automatic tools are more economical, since only part of the kit is disposable. However, the disadvantage is the lower control over the progression of the needle during discharge and capture of the fragment as well as the longer procedure time due to the increase in the number of preparation steps of the needle/spring-loaded tool with the risk of contamination. Semi-automatic tools are more costly due to the fact that the entire system is disposable. The advantages are the security in maintaining all material sterile throughout all steps of the procedure, greater control over the advancing of the needle for the extraction of the fragment, the possibility of checking the intralesional position prior to discharge, and the reduction in procedure time, since no preparation of the needle and spring-loaded tool is needed.

Prior to presenting the biopsy technique to the patient or legal guardian, it is advisable to consult with the physician in charge of the procedure. This moment orientates the patient and family regarding the risks, benefits, and preparation for the procedure. It is also possible to identify possible techniques linked to the peculiarities of each patient, such as having a physical disability that precludes the standard position, deforming kyphoscoliosis, scars, skin diseases, and anxiety disorders. To ensure a successful examination, it is of extreme importance to evaluate recent laboratory exams (within the previous 30 days) and determine the patient's health condition. Patients should meet basic criteria before being submitted to the procedure (**Table 1**). If a patient does not meet the minimum requirements, the procedure should be rescheduled until after the base disorder has been corrected. For patients with an urgent need for the procedure, immediate corrective measures should be assessed. For instance, plasma and platelet transfusion may be options in cases of a high international normalized ratio (INR) and low platelet count, respectively. An imaging study should be performed prior to the kidney biopsy to gain knowledge on renal anatomy and determine the presence of ectopias, congenital dysplasia, or polycystic kidneys.

2.3 Quality of material/pathologist present

A kidney biopsy is an important diagnostic tool and considered the "gold standard" for the best definition of the majority of nephropathies. It is capable of changing the clinical diagnosis approximately 50% of the time and changing the therapy to be administered approximately 40% of the time [16]. For this to happen, however, an adequate sample must be obtained.

A 19-gauge needle generally furnishes very small, narrow specimens that are often inadequate for the assessment of vessels. Thus, smaller needles, such as 18 or

Criteria that impede a kidney biopsy
Clotting disorders characterized by prothrombin activity <60%
INR > 1.3
Platelet count <60,000/mm^3
Use of anticoagulant
Systolic BP > 140 mm Hg
Urinary infection
Acute persistent cough
Skin lesions at puncture site
Altered mental state

Table 1.
Conditions that impede a kidney biopsy.

16 gauge, are advisable [17, 18]. Depending on the needle used, the difference in the obtainment of glomeruli can be as high as 300% [19]. The quantity of glomeruli needed for a secure diagnosis depends mainly on the diagnostic hypothesis and the clinical condition of the patient. For virtual exclusion (with greater than 95% certainty) of the diagnosis of focal segmental glomerulosclerosis, it is essential to have at least 25 glomeruli representing the juxtamedullary portion, as the focal disease affects some glomeruli while sparing others of morphological abnormalities seen with light microscopy and a good sample is important to the best definition of the disease [20]. In contrast, the diagnosis can be confirmed with a single glomerulus for other diseases, such as membranous glomerulopathy, in which diffuse morphological changes are similar in all glomeruli. For still other diseases, such as myeloma nephropathy, the diagnosis is essentially confirmed with representation of the medullary portion. In the analysis of transplanted kidney tissue, the aim is to achieve at least two core fragments exhibiting at least 7–10 glomeruli, two arteries, and the medullary portion (minimum assessment criteria defined by the Banff Meeting) [21].

In the evaluation of most glomerulopathies by light microscopy or immunofluorescence microscopy, 8–10 glomeruli are needed [22]. During the US-guided removal of the fragment, the evaluation of a pathologist is very important, as he/she is capable of determining the adequacy of the sample. The examination of the fresh material determines its sufficiency (quantity of glomeruli) for testing the main clinical hypotheses and provides information on medullary representation as well as the representation of larger vessels (**Figure 1**).

After determining the ideal amount of material and its representation of the renal parenchyma, the pathologist stores the samples in specific solutions for different analyses. The solutions should not come into contact with each other, as this would render the subsequent analyses unviable. The largest portion of the fragments should be allocated to light microscopy analysis. The most widely used fixatives are

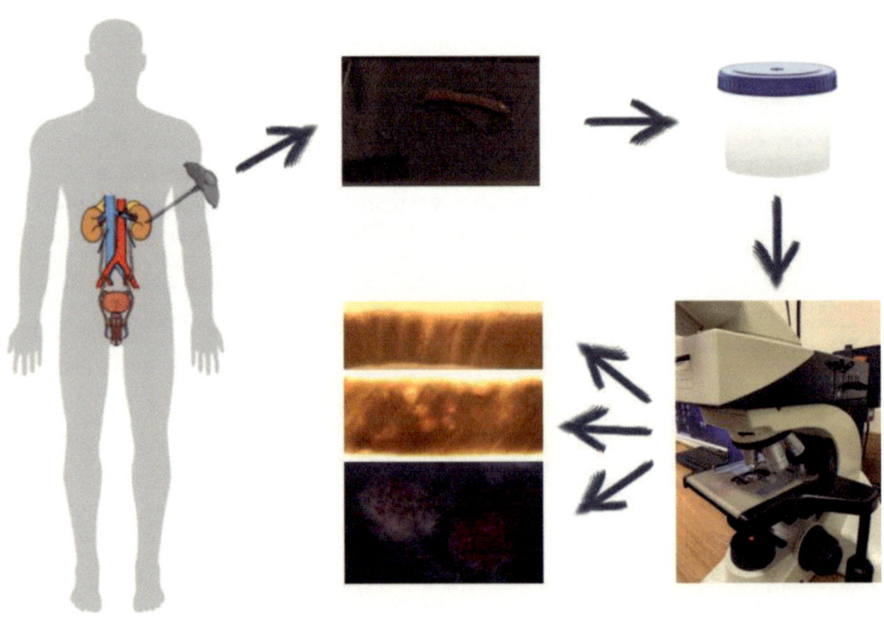

Figure 1.
Ultrasound-guided kidney biopsy. Fragment stored in 0.9% NaCl and analyzed under a light microscope. Renal medulla with medullary rays and characteristic striation. Multiple small round structures (glomeruli) distributed in renal cortex—some paler, others congested with numerous red blood cells (details of two glomerular structures).

10% neutral buffered formalin, paraformaldehyde, and Bouin's solution. In these media, the sample remains viable for analysis for several days. However, earlier histological processing results in analyses of better quality. For the analysis of antigens, such as IgG, IgM, IgA, complement components C3 and Cq1, fibrinogen as well as κ and λ chains, immunofluorescence microscopy should be used. Therefore, the sample should be stored in 0.9% saline solution—if the collection site is near the analysis site—and kept chilled (but not frozen) to obtain the best possible results. If rapid analysis (within several hours) is not possible, the sample should be placed in a transport solution, such as Michel's or Zeus solution. Although this solution preserves the sample for several days, better results are achieved the earlier the sample is taken for analysis, with poor or even impossible results if the sample is analyzed 5–7 days after being collected [23]. For transmission electron microscopy, a small portion is needed of the cortical parenchyma, with two glomeruli. This analysis is essential to the evaluation of podocytopathies, thin basement membrane disease, and metabolic disease. The fragments should be fixed within minutes after collection in a specific solution (glutaraldehyde or Karnovsky's solution). In the presence of a pathologist, a small portion may be acquired (1 and 2 mm) and fragmented until obtaining the quantity of glomeruli needed. This material should be placed in a buffered solution after fixation (1–2 days after collection), as the aim of the analysis is to examine the ultrastructure, such as the cytoplasmic membrane, reticulum, and immune deposits, which are lost if not fixed soon enough.

When a biopsy is performed without the presence of a nephropathologist, it is advisable to remove at least one fragment (if possible, two) from the renal parenchyma for each solution. Immunohistochemical analysis for the study of C4d, polyomavirus, adenovirus, cytomegalovirus, PLA2R, IgG4, etc. should be performed with material embedded in paraffin, which is preserved for light microscopy.

2.4 Complications and management

A kidney biopsy is considered a minimally invasive method but is not without complications. Depending on the severity, such events are classified as minor and major, which require different forms of treatment (**Table 2**). Minor complications include hematuria, small perirenal hematomas, arteriovenous fistulas, and pain, all of which normally resolve spontaneously [24]. Major complications include massive bleeding with hemodynamic instability, voluminous perirenal hematomas with refractory disabling pain, and important hematuria with obstruction of the urinary tract by clots. In such cases, management is normally necessary.

Among all forms of complication, bleeding is the most frequent and occurs mainly within the first 12–24 hours after the procedure in nearly all patients [4, 25].

Complications	**Management**
Major complications	
Disabling intense pain	Optimization of analgesia (use of opioids)
Hemodynamic instability with blood transfusion	Endovascular treatment (embolization)
Clot obstructing urinary tract	Irrigation with three-way probe
Minor complications	
Arteriovenous fistula	Conservative
Hematuria	Hydration

Table 2.
Post-biopsy complication and proper management for each.

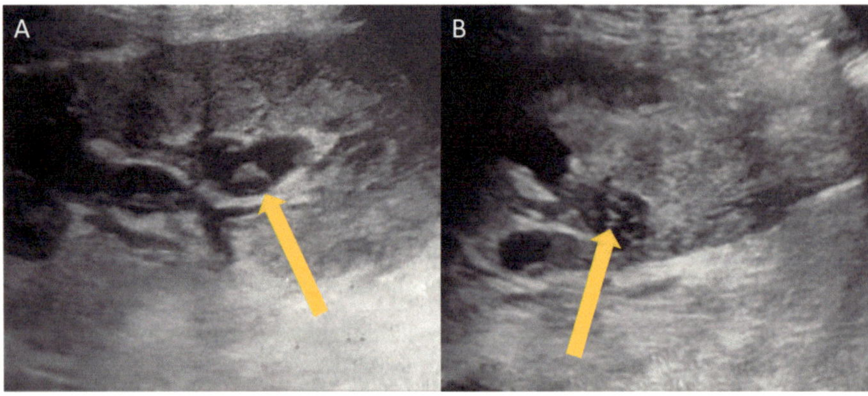

Figure 2.
Exploratory ultrasound performed on patient with gross hematuria, 24 hours after percutaneous native kidney biopsy. (A and B) Multiple pelvic blood clots (arrow) after renal biopsy.

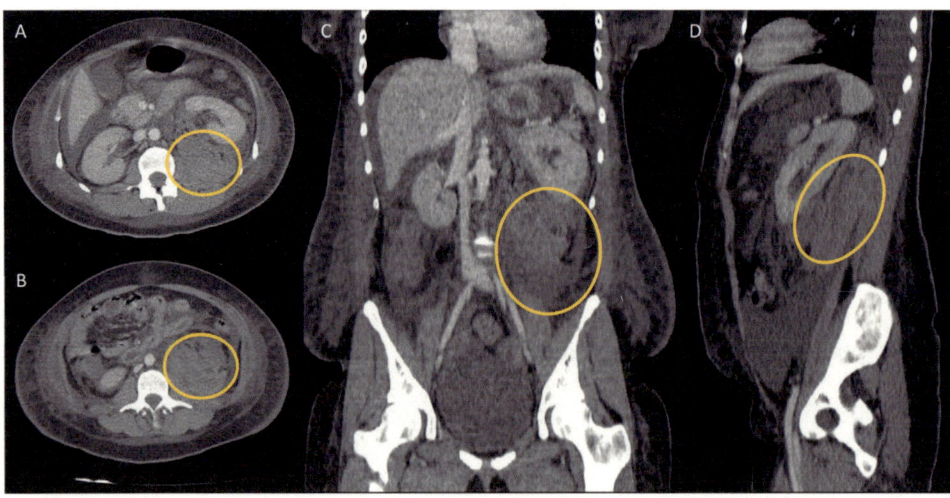

Figure 3.
Perirenal hematoma, an hour after percutaneous native kidney biopsy. Computed tomography (CT) scan slices of the abdomen revealed voluminous perirenal hematoma (yellow circle), on the left side. (A and B) Axial scan slices. (C) Coronal scan slice. (D) Coronal scan slice.

Microscopic hematuria, mild low back pain, and a slight drop in the hemoglobin concentration are frequent findings and should not be considered complications [25]. However, the persistence of these symptoms for more than a week may require a detailed investigation with imaging exams. Post-biopsy chronic hypertension, the puncture of other organs, and perirenal soft part infections have been described but are very rare.

The literature reports variable complication rates, generally ranging from 5 to 16%, with macroscopic hematuria in 3–9% of cases and the need for transfusions in 0.1–3.0% of cases [14, 26–29]. In such cases, an exploratory ultrasound examination should be performed (**Figure 2**). Burstein et al. found post-biopsy complications in 14.3% of patients, with 6.6% considered minor and another 7.7% considered major (hemorrhages requiring blood transfusion or another approach) [28]. González-Michaca et al. found major complications in 2.4% of patients and minor complications in 8.65%, the most frequent of which was perirenal hematoma [30, 31]. Native kidneys tend to have a lower complication rate than transplanted kidneys (13.9 and 24.4%, respectively) [32].

DOI: http://dx.doi.org/10.5772/intechopen.89226

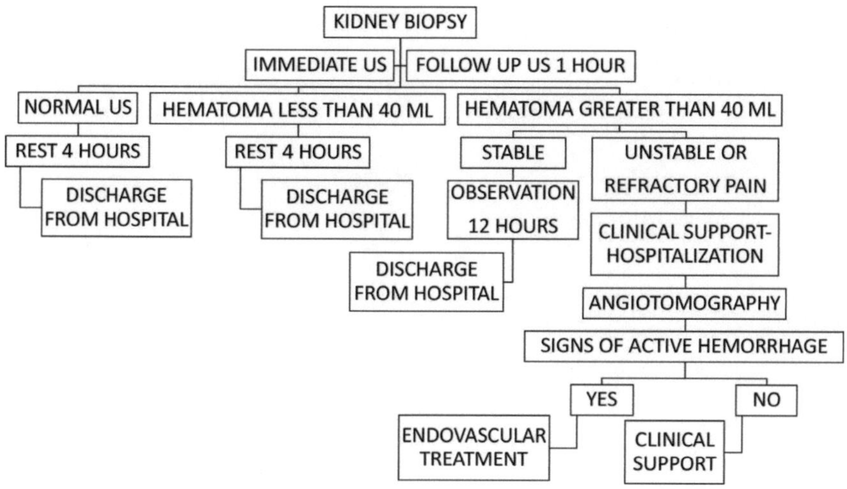

Figure 4.
Post-biopsy procedures and management.

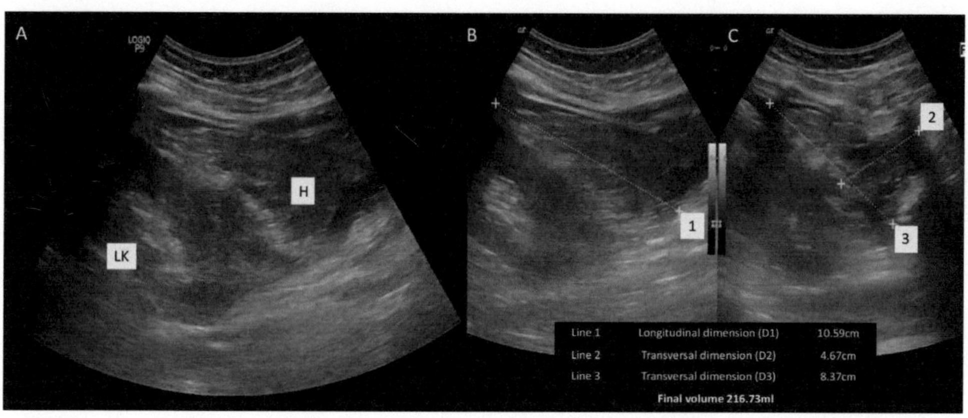

Figure 5.
Perirenal hematoma, observed an hour after percutaneous native kidney biopsy. (A) Longitudinal ultrasonography exhibiting hematoma area near the posteroinferior border of the left kidney. (B and C) Longitudinal (line 1) and transversal dimension on ultrasound (line 2 and 3) estimated the final volume of 216.73 ml of hematoma area. LK, left kidney; H, hematoma.

After a kidney biopsy, patients should remain in observation for at least 4 hours. They are placed at absolute rest in dorsal decubitus and are monitored in this period with the constant evaluation of vital signs. It is also advisable to perform renal ultrasound 1 hour after the procedure in all patients submitted to percutaneous kidney biopsy. The aim of this measure is to evaluate the biopsied area and anticipate possible post-procedure complications, thereby enabling immediate, effective therapeutic support (**Figure 3** and **Figure 4**).

The volume of the perirenal hematoma formed and the complication rates associated with this procedure have a direct relation of proportionality. Hematomas formed in the first hour after the procedure with volumes greater than 40 ml are related to a greater risk of developing major complications [14] (**Figure 5**). For cases of minor complications, the patient should receive clear orientation regarding the expected benign evolution of the case and receive medication for the symptoms based on individual need. These patients should be required to return after 7 days for a follow-up ultrasound and definitive discharge of the case if no imaging abnormalities are found and there are no new complaints. In cases of hemodynamic

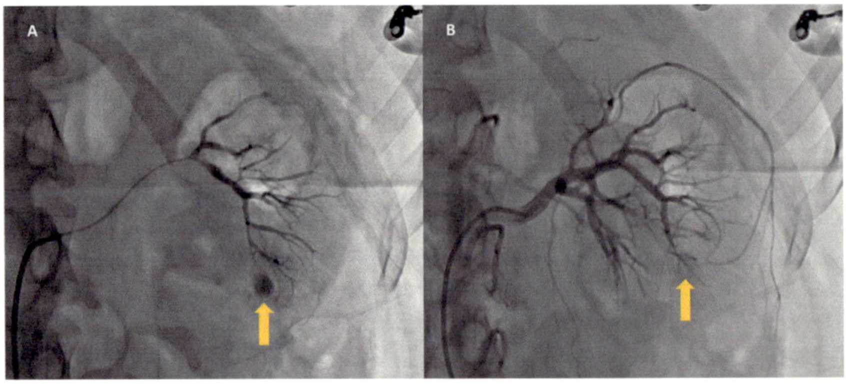

Figure 6.
Renal arteriography, 2 hours after percutaneous native kidney biopsy. (A) Pre-embolization arteriography revealed pseudoaneurysm in a lower renal pole (yellow arrow). (B) Post-embolization superselective arteriography revealed absence of pseudoaneurysm with preservation of the local vasculature (yellow arrow).

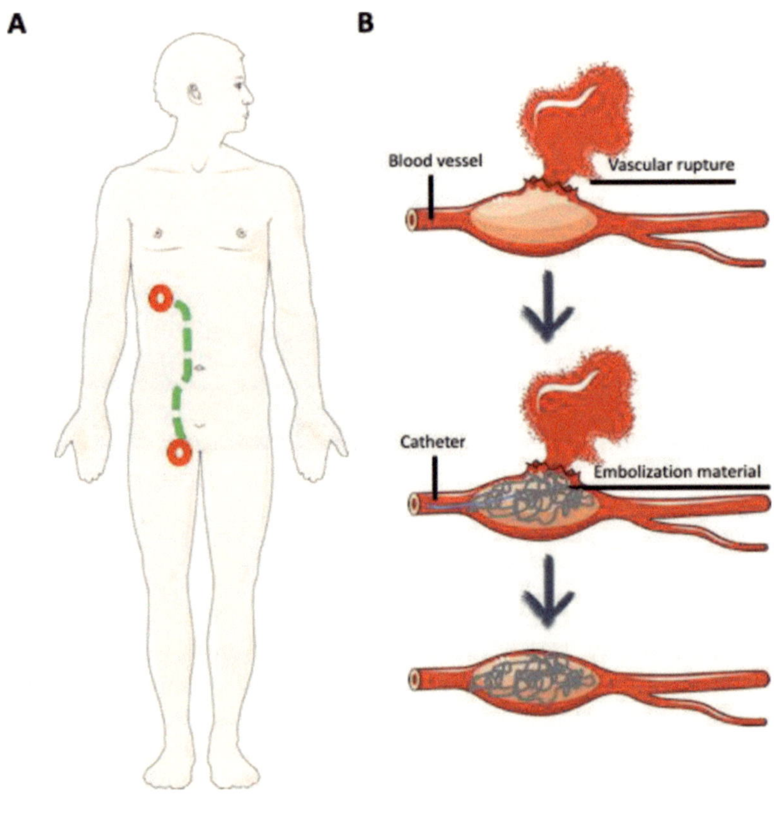

Figure 7.
Endovascular embolization. (A) A catheter is inserted into femoral artery, by the groin area to access vessels of the kidney and into vascular rupture site. (B) Rupture in arterial blood vessel, which will receive a catheter and embolization material to achieve occlusion.

instability, the patient should receive adequate clinical measures at an intensive care unit, followed by an angiographic study. Digital angiography remains the gold standard for the anatomic study of the renal arteries, but computed tomography angiography (angiotomography) has gained popularity, offering comparable accuracy and the advantage of evaluating not only the lumen, but its walls and other visceral changes [32].

After renal vascular mapping and if signs of active bleeding are identified (active escape of contrast medium, pseudoaneurysms, or arteriovenous fistulas), endovascular treatment is indicated, which is a minimally invasive procedure that should be performed by an interventionist radiologist or professional who is duly trained and certified in endovascular techniques (**Figure 6**). The procedure can be performed through femoral or radial artery access, always initiated with an anatomic study of the renal arteries and respective variations. When a probable focal hemorrhage is identified, superselective arteriography is performed in a coaxial system with a microcatheter and microguide, followed by superselective embolization techniques performed on the compromised vessel. For interventional treatment, the selection of appropriate embolic agents for superselective embolization is the key to achieving desirable outcomes (**Figure 7**). Embolic agents include PVA particles, coils, and gelatin sponge strips, which can be used either alone or in combination [33]. The de-vascularized area will suffer infarction, which could cause a momentary change in renal function. Thus, more selective catheterism leads to a lower risk of this complication. Pseudoaneurysms are pulsating masses at puncture sites due to the rupture of the arterial wall and extravasation of blood, generally associated with local pain and hematoma. Hemodynamic instability and a drop in hemoglobin concentration may be related to the rupture of pseudoaneurysms. The treatment for pseudoaneurysms and arteriovenous fistulas is recommended for persistent bleeding for more than 72 hours or in cases of the accentuated loss of kidney function after the procedure. It should be stressed that most pseudoaneurysms less than 2.0 cm and arteriovenous fistulas progress with thrombosis and spontaneous resolution within 4 weeks, making conservative treatment the conduct of choice in cases without hemodynamic instability. Patients should remain in intensive care for at least 24 hours after the procedure and a follow-up imaging method should be performed prior to the decision regarding the discharge of these patients.

3. Conclusion

Imaging-guided renal biopsy is a useful tool for the evaluation and management of renal diseases. This chapter summarizes that percutaneous ultrasound-guided renal biopsy is a safe technique which allows the evaluation of renal disease but is associated with post-biopsy complications. We discuss indications and approach to imaging-guided percutaneous renal biopsies as well as complications and management associated with this.

Acknowledgements

We thank Instituto de Ensino e Pesquisa da Santa Casa de Belo Horizonte, Hospital Santa Casa de Belo Horizonte, Brazil and Coordenação de Aperfeiçoamento de Pessoal de Nível Superior (CAPES), Brazil.

Conflict of interest

The authors declare no conflict of interest.

Author details

Paulo Ramos Botelho Antunes[1,2], Stanley Almeida Araújo[3], Silvana Maria Carvalho Miranda[4,5], Fabiano Franco Monteiro Prado[1,2], Luiz Felipe França Antunes[1,2], Elisa Carvalho de Siqueira[1], Fabrício Tinôco Alvim de Souza[1*] and Maria Carolina Barbosa Álvares[1,2]

1 Research Group on Diagnostic and Therapeutic Radiology, Santa Casa de Belo Horizonte, Belo Horizonte, Brazil

2 Diagnostic and Therapeutic Radiology Service, Santa Casa de Belo Horizonte, Belo Horizonte, Brazil

3 Institute of Nephropathology, Federal University of Minas Gerais, Belo Horizonte, Brazil

4 Nephrology Service, Santa Casa de Belo Horizonte, Belo Horizonte, Brazil

5 Transplant Service, Santa Casa de Belo Horizonte, Belo Horizonte, Brazil

*Address all correspondence to: ftadesouza@gmail.com

References

[1] Makris K, Spanou L. Acute kidney injury: Definition, pathophysiology and clinical phenotypes. Clinical Biochemist Reviews. 2016;**37**(2):85-98

[2] Ferenbach DA, Bonventre JV. Acute kidney injury and chronic kidney disease: From the laboratory to the clinic. Néphrologie and Thérapeutique. 2016;**12**(1):S41-S48. DOI: 10.1016/j.nephro.2016.02.005

[3] Bandari J, Fuller TW, Turner RM II, D'Agostino LA. Renal biopsy for medical renal disease: Indications and contraindications. The Canadian Journal of Urology. 2016;**23**(1):8121-8126

[4] Luciano RL, Moeckel GW. Update on the native kidney biopsy: Core curriculum 2019. American Journal of Kidney Diseases. 2019;**73**(3):404-415. DOI: 10.1053/j.ajkd.2018.10.011

[5] Hogan JJ, Mocanu M, Bernes JS. The native kidney biopsy: Update and evidence for best practice. Clinical Journal of the American Society of Nephrology. 2016;**11**(2):354-362

[6] Whittier WL, Korbet SM. Indications for and Complications of Renal Biopsy. In: UpToDate, Post TW, editors. Waltham, MA: UpToDate; 2019

[7] Lefaucheur C, Nochy D, Bariety J. Bopsie renale: Techniques de prélèvement, contre-indications, complications renal biopsy: Procedures, contraindications, complications. Néphrologie and Thérapeutique. 2009;**5**(4):331-339. DOI: 10.1016/j.nephro.2009.02.005

[8] Alshami A, Roshan A, Catapang M, Jöbsis JJ, Kwok T, Polderman N, et al. Pediatric nephrology clinical pathway development team. Indications for kidney biopsy in idiopathic childhood nephrotic syndrome. Pediatric Nephrology. 2017;**32**(10):1897-1905. DOI: 10.1007/s00467-017-3687-3

[9] Richards NT, Darby S, Howie AJ, Adu D, Michael J. Knowledge of renal histology alters patient management in over 40% of cases. Nephrology, Dialysis, Transplantation. 1994;**9**(9):1255-1259

[10] Gulati S, Sharma AP, Sharma RK, Gupta A, Gupta RK. Do current recommendations for kidney biopsy in nephrotic syndrome need modifications? Pediatric Nephrology. 2002;**17**:404-408. DOI: 10.1007/s00467-002-0840-3

[11] Nammalwar BR, Vijayakumar M, Prahlad N. Experience of renal biopsy in children with nephrotic syndrome. Pediatric Nephrology. 2006;**21**:286-288. DOI: 10.1007/s00467-005-2084-5

[12] Ali H, Murtaza A, Anderton J, Ahmed A. Post renal biopsy complication rate and diagnostic yield comparing hands free (ultrasound-assisted) and ultrasound-guided biopsy techniques of renal allografts and native kidneys. Springerplus. 2015;**4**(1):491. DOI: 10.1186/s40064-015-1292-0

[13] Rivera Gorrín M, Correa Gorospe C, Burguera V, Ortiz Chercoles AI, Liaño F, Quereda C. Teaching innovations in ultrasound-guided renal biopsy. Nefrología. 2016;**36**(1):1-4. DOI: 10.1016/j.nefro.2015.07.011

[14] Antunes PRB, Prado FFM, de Souza FTA, de Siqueira EC, de Campos MÁ, Álvares MCB, et al. Clinical complications in renal biopsy using two different needle gauges: The impact of large hematomas, a random clinical trial study. International Journal of Urology. 2018;**25**(6):544-548. DOI: 10.1111/iju.13559

[15] Hatfield MK, Beres RA, Sane SS, Zaleski GX. Percutaneous imaging-guided solid organ core needle biopsy: Coaxial versus noncoaxial

method. AJR. American Journal of Roentgenology. 2008;**190**(2):413-417. DOI: 10.2214/AJR.07.2676

[16] Fogo AB, Cohen AH, Colvin RB, Jennette JC, Alpers CE. Fundamentals of Renal Pathology. 2nd ed. Berlin: Springer; 2014. 230p

[17] Corwin HL, Schwartz MM, Lewis EJ. The importance of sample size in the interpretation of the renal biopsy. American Journal of Nephrology. 1988;**8**(2):85-89. DOI: 10.1159/000167563

[18] Oberholzer M, Torhorst E, Perret E, Mihatsch MJ. Minimum sample size of kidney biopsies for semiquantitative and quantitative evaluation. Nephron. 1983;**34**(3):192-195. DOI: 10.1159/000183008

[19] Mostbeck GH, Wittich GR, Derfler K, Ulrich W, Walter RM, Herold C, et al. Optimal needle size for renal biopsy: In vitro and in vivo evaluation. Radiology. 1989;**173**(3):819-822. DOI: 10.1148/radiology.173.3.2813792

[20] Fogo AB. Core curriculum in nephrology—Approach to renal biopsy. American Journal of Kidney Diseases. 2003;**42**(4):826-836

[21] Racusen LC, Solez K, Colvin RB, Bonsib SM, Castro MC, Cavallo T, et al. The Banff 97 working classification of renal allograft pathology. Kidney International. 1999;**55**(2):713-723. DOI: 10.1046/j.1523-1755.1999.00299.x

[22] Working Group of the International IgA Nephropathy Network and the Renal Pathology Society, Cattran DC, Coppo R, Cook HT, Feehally J, Roberts IS, et al. The Oxford classification of IgA nephropathy: Rationale, clinicopathological correlations, and classification. Kidney International. 2009;**76**(5):534-545. DOI: 10.1038/ki.2009.243

[23] Michel B, Milner Y, David K. Preservation of tissue-fixed immunoglobulins in skin biopsies of patients with lupus erythematosus and bullous diseases—Preliminary report. The Journal of Investigative Dermatology. 1972;**59**(6):449-452

[24] Korbet SM. Percutaneous renal biopsy. Seminars in Nephrology. 2002;**22**(3):254-267. DOI: 10.2214/AJR.07.2676

[25] Carnevale FC. Tratado de radiologia intervencionista e cirurgia endovascular. 1st ed. Rio de Janeiro: Thieme Revinter Publicações; 2017. 1216p

[26] Tøndel C, Vikse BE, Bostad L, Svarstad E. Safety and complications of percutaneous kidney biopsies in 715 children and 8573 adults in Norway 1988-2010. Clinical Journal of the American Society of Nephrology. 2012;7(10):1591-1597. DOI: 10.2215/CJN.02150212

[27] Choi IJ, Jeong HJ, Han DS, Lee JS, Choi KH, Kang SW, et al. An analysis of 4.514 cases of renal biopsies in Korea. Yonsei Medical Journal. 2001;**42**(2):247-254. DOI: 10.3349/ymj.2001.42.2.247

[28] Burstein D, Korbet S, Schwartz M. The use of the automated core biopsy system in percutaneous renal biopsies. A comparative study. American Journal of Kidney Diseases. 1993;**22**:545-552

[29] Wickre CG, Golper TA. Complications of percutaneos needle biopsy of the kidney. American Journal of Nephrology. 1982;**2**:173-178. DOI: 10.1159/00016664030

[30] González-Michaca L, Chew-Wong A, Soltero L, Gamba G, Correa-Rotter R. Percutaneous kidney biopsy, analysis of 26 years: Complication rate and risk factors. Revista de Investigación Clínica. 2000;**52**(2):125-131

[31] Lasmar EP. Biopsia renal percutânea: experiência pessoal em 30 anos. Jornal Brasileiro de Nefrologia. 2007;**29**:25-28

[32] Peynircioğlu B, Pişkinkaya S, Özer Ç, Çil B, Yorgancıoğlu C, Arıcı M. Isolated spontaneous renal artery dissection: Diagnosis and endovascular management. Diagnostic and Interventional Radiology. 2011;**17**(1):101-104. DOI: 10.4261/1305-3825.DIR.2786-09.1

[33] Wang HL, Xu CY, Wang HH, Xu W. Emergency transcatheter arterial embolization for acute renal hemorrhage. Medicine (Baltimore). 2015;**94**(42):e1667. DOI: 10.1097/MD.0000000000001667

Chapter 6

Causes and Pathophysiology of Nephrotic Syndrome in Childhood

Nagaraju Vallepu, Saikiran Velpula, Bharath Kumar Dasari, Manish Kumar Thimmaraju, Sridhar Babu Gummadi, Neeraja Yelugam and Supraja Jannu

Abstract

Nephrotic syndrome is a general type of kidney disease seen in children. In the past, Roelans is credited with the first clinical description of nephrotic syndrome in the late fifteenth century. Nephrotic syndrome is appropriate to excessive hypoalbuminemia, edema, and proteinuria may be hyperlipidemia also present in some cases. Periorbital swelling with or without edema of the body is observed in first starting little period of life, frequently show in children with this condition. Nephrotic syndrome starts develops due functional and structural changes in the GFB, consequential difficulty to control protein in the urine. Nephrotic syndrome possibly causes due to some of glomerular diseases and systemic diseases, but significantly the mostly in childhood is unknown nephrotic syndrome. The first significant improvement with introduction of sulfonamides and then penicillin was seen in 1939. The beginning of adrenocorticotropic hormone and cortisone greater decrease in mortality (to 9%), in the 1950s it was noted to happen in association with spectacular declaration of proteinuria. Etiology of nephrotic syndrome is also age reliant. Most cases reported in the first 3 months of life are referred to as congenital nephrotic syndrome (CNS) and are due to genetic diseases.

Keywords: nephrotic syndrome, hypoalbuminemia, proteinuria, glomerular filtration barrier, congenital nephrotic syndrome

1. Introduction

Nephrotic syndrome is a general type of kidney disease seen in children. Historically, Roelans is credited with the first clinical description of nephrotic syndrome in the late fifteenth century. Nephrotic syndrome is appropriate to excessive hypoalbuminemia, proteinuria, and edema, although additional clinical hyperlipidemia is also usually present. The beginning of adrenocorticotropic hormone and cortisone in the 1950s contributed to an even greater decrease in mortality (to 9%), which was noted to occur in association with dramatic resolution of proteinuria.

2. Causes

The childhood nephrotic syndrome is principally idiopathic or primary, though a limited number of cases are secondary to glomerular and inclusive diseases and other infectious agents. Age reliant is also the etiology factor of nephrotic syndrome. Maximum cases presenting in the first 3 months of lifespan are mentioned as CNS (congenital nephrotic syndrome) and are caused by genetic diseases. While in the remaining of the first year of lifecycle (3–12 months) there has been no effective study of the etiology of nephrotic syndrome reported cases, there are a number of stats shows that up to 40% of reported cases meanwhile this time may also be due to genetic factors [1]. At the time of first year and in the first decade of life, maximum presenting cases are due to primary or idiopathic nephrotic syndrome, at the time of first 10 years of lifecycle the number of secondary nephrotic syndrome cases increases.

2.1 Inborn nephrotic syndrome

Congenital nephrotic syndrome is the type of nephrotic syndrome which occurs in first 3 months of life and is due to genetic causes mostly by alterations in the gene encrypting nephrin, a podocyte opening diaphragm protein. For the first time, these mutations were expressed in the Finnish, from then the name congenital nephrotic syndrome of the Finnish type (CNF) [1]. Though the incidence of CNF is high in Finland it also occurs in other populations also. Congenital nephrotic syndrome is not either equivalent with CNF, reason is that alterations in other genes encrypting podocyte opening diaphragm proteins, early-onset nephrotic syndrome can also be caused by proteins such as podocin. Upto 40% of all cases of nephrotic syndrome occurring in the first 3 months of life are due to alterations in a sequence of podocin gene [2] in the earliest 3 months of life. Nephrotic syndrome may also be part of multisystemic syndromes such as nail-patella syndrome, Pierson syndrome, Denys-Drash syndrome, and others or a sequence of congenital infections such as cytomegalovirus and syphilis (**Table 1**).

Genetic	Mutation in nephrin *(NPHS1)* gene leads to congenital nephrotic syndrome of the Finnish type (CNF) Mutation in podocin *(NPHS2)* gene results Autosomal recessive FSGS Mutation in *WT1* gene results Autosomal dominant diffuse mesangial Sclerosis (DMS) Mutation in laminin β_2 gene leads Congenital nephrotic syndrome
Syndromes	Nail-patella syndrome due to mutation in LIM homeodomain protein (LMX1B) Jeune's syndrome Galloway Mowat syndrome Denys-Drash syndrome due to WT1 mutation with DMS Pierson syndrome Schimke immunoosseous dysplasia with FSGS due to mutation in SMARCAL1 Cockayne syndrome
Idiopathic	Nonsyndromic DMS Minimal change nephrotic syndrome FSGS
Infections	Congenital toxoplasmosis Congenital cytomegalovirus (CMV) infection Congenital syphilis

Table 1.
Causative factors of congenital nephrotic syndrome (CNS) in 0–3 months of age.

2.2 Nephrotic syndrome after infancy

Above the infancy and above the first year of life, maximum of the nephrotic syndrome cases are idiopathic. MCNS (Minimal-Change Nephrotic Syndrome) is the most usual deviation, and is responsible for more than 80% of all cases [3]. Focal segmental glomerulosclerosis (FSGS), Membranoproliferative glomerulonephritis (MPGN), and mesangial multiply glomerulonephritis are the other less common histopathologic types in this age group (**Table 2**). For a few cases in this age group genetic disease is also responsible. 10–25% of all cases of familial and sporadic SRNS were caused by

Idiopathic	C1q nephropathy IgM nephropathy Membranous nephropathy (MN) Membranoproliferative glomerulonephritis (MPGN) Minimal change nephrotic syndrome (MCNS) Focal segmental glomerulosclerosis (FSGS) Mesangial proliferative glomerulonephritis
Hereditary	Mutation in *WT1* gene results autosomal dominant diffuse mesangial Sclerosis (DMS) Mutation in gene encoding transient receptor potential cation channel 6 *(TRPC6)* results Autosomal dominant FSGS Mutation in gene encoding CD2-associated protein *(CD2AP)* results autosomal dominant FSGS Mutation in gene encoding *α-actinin 4* leads to autosomal dominant FSGS Mutation in podocin*(NPHS2)* gene results autosomal recessive FSGS
Drugs	NSAIDs Penicillamine ACEIs Pamidronate Gold Lithium Mercury Interferon Heroin
Metabolic diseases	Glutaric acidemia Mitochondrial cytopathies Glycogen storage disease Fabry's disease
General diseases	Systemic lupus erythematosus Sarcoidosis Diabetes mellitus Henoch-Schönlein purpura
Blood and oncologic diseases	Lymphoma (Hodgkin's most likely can lead to minimal change) Leukemia Sickle cell disease
Infections	HIV Malaria Filariasis Schistosomiasis Hepatitis B and C
Others	Food allergies Obesity (usually with FSGS) Bee stings (MCNS) Pregnancy Oligomeganephronia

Table 2.
Causative factors of nephrotic syndrome above 3 months of life.

mutations in NPHS2, inherited in an autosomal genetic mode, because it was exposed in one series. Beginning of nephrotic syndrome in untimely childhood, not response to steroid treatment, strong findings of focal segmental glomerulosclerosis (FSGS) on histopathology renal biopsy, progress to ESRD in 5 years of finding, and comprehensively decreases the risk of disease recurrence following renal transplantation are by the phenotype typically associated with NPHS2 mutations [4, 5]. Additional genetic factors consists autosomal dominant transmitted causes such as α-actinin 4, mutations in the Wilms' tumor suppressor gene (WT1), TRPC6 and CD2AP [6–10]. Individually from those in WT1, maximum of these mutations go to result in adult-onset disease. To a number of systemic diseases in children, nephrotic syndrome may also be secondary. Pediatric diseases such as Henoch-Schönlein purpura; diabetes mellitus; systemic lupus erythematosus, especially membranous (WHO Class V) SLE; and sarcoidosis may all exist with nephrotic syndrome. Infective factors can also cause nephrotic syndrome and can be bacterial, viral, or parasitic. Despite it is not so far fully known how these factors cause nephrotic syndrome, it is maybe due to an bizarre immune response to them in the majority of the reported cases, occurring in the progression and aggregation of immune complexes in the glomerulus. The interpretation of these factors as a cause of nephrotic syndrome turn to parallel their prevalence in demanding regions of the world. For example, in Hong Kong and countries in Africa, hepatitis B and C are important causes of nephrotic syndrome [11, 12]. In areas where malaria is endemic, Malaria, particularly quartan malaria, is also an important cause. Eighteen nephrotic syndrome in both adults and children can be caused by Human immunodeficiency virus (HIV).despite the renal abrasion linked with HIV can be changeable, FSGS is the most common histologic finding affiliated with HIV is, particularly the breakdown is different. Despite the result of treatment of the underlying infection on the nephropathy is not well known, but there are details that hepatitis B-associated nephrotic syndrome may be cooperative to treatment of the hepatitis [13]. A list of infective factors associated with nephrotic syndrome is shown in **Table 2**. Drugs such as angiotensin converting enzyme inhibitors (ACEIs), penicillamine, gold, nonsteroidal antiinflammatory drugs (NSAIDs), sickle cell disease, bee stings, lymphoma, leukemia, and various types of food allergies are the other less common causes of nephrotic syndrome. Moreover, in children with obesity the nephrotic syndrome is being seen further recurrently. The histologic scrape most frequently occurs in this setting is FSGS.

3. Mechanism of nephrotic syndrome

The development of massive proteinuria is the central abnormality in all cases of nephrotic syndrome. Some of the literature shows the evidence in that nephrotic syndrome may be a significance of glomerular defect, circulating factors, and defect in immunological system.

3.1 Glomerular defect

The most important possible functions of the kidney is the filtration of blood and blood products at glomeruli, which permits the fluid and dirty products while retaining the greater part of blood proteins and all blood cells within the vasculature. These types of process of filtration is made potential by the (GFB), which is made up of specific glomerular epithelial cells (podocytes), endothelial cells, and GBM these distal bottom actions are attached to the GBM (**Figure 1**) [14]. Adjacent podocyte bottom actions are associated to each one other by networks of specific cell-cell junctions called as opening diaphragms. Additionally, the GBM (glomerular basement membrane) has a plentiful supplies of negatively charged molecules of heparin sulfate

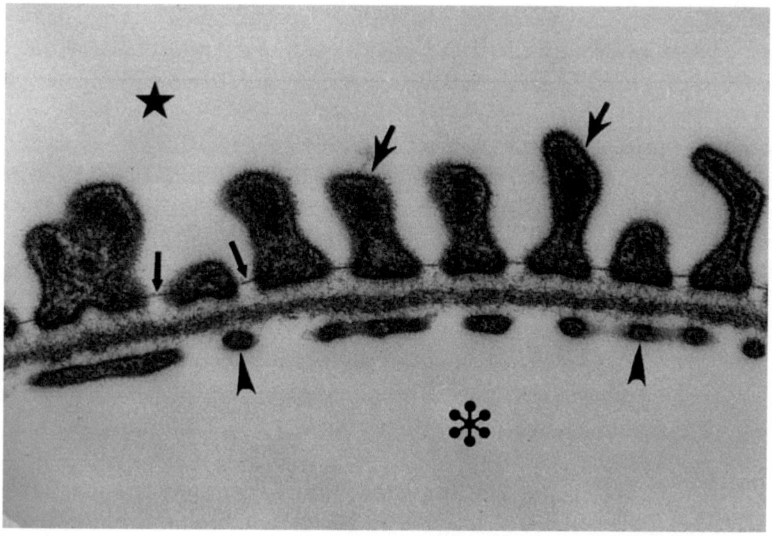

Figure 1.
Components of the glomerular filtration barrier (GFB) during normal glomerular filtration, electron micrographic view.

proteoglycan, resultant in these negatively charged heparin sulfate proteoglycan controlled from passage than positively charged molecules with same particles [15]. General healthy system, particle more than 42 Å in diameter is not capable to enter into the GFB [16]. This kind of restrictions based on mostly structural reliability of the podocyte bottom actions and opening diaphragms, by means of the charge of GBM. Loss of negative charge of the GBM occurs in nephrotic syndrome [17–19]. The confirmation, swelling and diffusion podocyte binds to bottom actions, dislocation of opening diaphragms, occurrence of filling junctions, vacuole formation, and deficiency of inclusion of podocytes from the GBM, these type of morphologic changes in podocytes that occur during progress of nephrotic syndrome [20–23]. Mutations in genes encoding some of the opening diaphragms proteins or their transcription factors can cause SRNS and/or FSGS. This mechanism of nephrotic syndrome is additional reinforced by recent observations in humans and experimental animals [4, 10, 11, 14, 24–26]. The subject of many recent reviews in the literature this type of result have been discussed [27–29]. In infants mutations in the gene encoding the opening diaphragms protein nephrin (NPHS1) mostly causes CNF. In addition, in children mutations in NPHS2 are estimated to be responsible for up to 25% of cases of sporadic familial and Steroid resistant nephrotic syndrome (SRNS) [10, 25]. Frasier syndrome and Denys rash syndrome in children occurs due to Mutations in the transcription factor suppressor gene WT1 [30–32]. Mutations in (1) CD2-associated protein (CD2AP); (2) the LIM-homeodomain protein (encoded by LMX1B), which leads to in nail-patella syndrome; (3) the actin-bundling protein α-actinin 4, which leads to adult-onset FSGS; which results in adult-onset FSGS; (4) laminin β2, which results in Pierson syndrome and (5) the chromatin regulator encoded by SMARCAL1. [25, 33–35].

3.2 Circulatory factors

Some of soluble mediators that may alter capillary wall permeability in nephrotic syndrome proved by investigational data to carry the existence [37–39] show to be true for this includes (1) scared decrease of proteinuria subsequent treatment with protein A immunoadsorption in of primary nephrotic syndromes [24], (2) progress of nephrotic syndrome in child babies born to mothers with nephrotic syndrome who actually transferred a soluble factor to their fetuses in utero [39], (3) decrease of repeated disease induced by treatment with protein A immunoadsorption due to presumed removal of circulating factors in the reappearance of FSGS in transplanted kidneys in patients with primary FSGS [40], and (4) FSGS recurrence in transplanted kidney patients serum injected in to the experimental animals leads to causing of enhanced glomerular permeability [32] serum of children with FSGS and recognized as components of apolipoproteins, from the suggestive of that an imbalance involving serum permeability factors and permeability inhibitors may have a pathogenic role in FSGS. Moreover, inhibitors of glomerular permeability have also been isolated [33].

3.3 Defect in immunological system

For more than 30 years nephrotic syndrome may be because of abnormalities of the immune system has existed. Both the humoral and cellular immune responses are abnormal during relapse of nephrotic syndrome. Still, have a thought that relationship between the nephrotic syndrome and T lymphocyte function was first proposed by Shalhoub and his colleagues and concluded that abnormalities in cellular immune responses [36] proves for this includes (1) sensitivity of most forms of primary nephrotic syndrome to mycophenolate mofetil, corticosteroids, calcineurin inhibitors, and alkylating agents, these drugs all are inhibitors of T lymphocyte purpose, (2) mostly measles and malaria, diseases well-known to slow down the cell-mediated immunity following remission of nephrotic syndrome, and (3) detection of Minimal-Change Nephrotic Syndrome (MCNS) as a paraneoplastic manifestation of lymphoreticular malignancies and other Hodgkin's disease. Latest reported cases have also suggested and vital role of the cell-mediated immune system in nephrotic syndrome, collectively with depressed cell-mediated immunity during relapses of MCNS alterations in T cell subsets during relapses and increased cell surface expression of IL-2 receptors on T cells, reflective of T cell activation [34, 41]. Additionally, a number of cytokines, released in part by T lymphocytes, have been recommended to be erratically changed throughout nephrotic syndrome (NS) [42, 43].

4. Pathophysiology

In children with nephrotic syndrome facial or general edema, is the basic symptom due to accumulation of fluid in the interstitial compartment. In nephrotic syndrome the edema is usually causes disproportionate proteinuria, which leads to retention of sodium and water, hypoalbuminemia to recompense for intravascular volume depletion. The pathogenesis of edema can be well explained by analysis of the classic Starling equation, which explains the regulation of fluid movement across capillary walls [44].

$$\text{Net filtration} = \text{LpS} \, (\Delta \text{ hydraulic pressure} - \Delta \text{ oncotic pressure}).$$

$$= \text{LpS} \, [(\text{Pcap} - \text{Pif}) - \text{s}(\pi\text{cap} - \pi\text{if})].$$

where:
Lp = the capillary permeability.
S = the surface area of the capillary wall.
Pcap = the capillary hydrostatic pressure.
Pif = the interstitial fluid hydrostatic fluid pressure.
s = the reflection coefficient for proteins (0 = complete permeability and 1 = complete impermeability).
πcap = the capillary oncotic pressure.
πif = the interstitial fluid oncotic pressure.

The formation of edema is prevented in healthy patients by a balance between forces favoring edema (capillary hydrostatic pressure [Pcap]) and those opposing it (capillary oncotic pressure [πcap]). The slight tendency toward fluid accumulation is counterbalanced by the lymphatics in the interstitial space. In nephrotic patients hypoalbuminemia results when the liver fails to synthesize the loss of albumin through urine. The hypoalbuminemia results leads to low down capillary oncotic pressure (πcap), which leads to relatively unopposed capillary hydrostatic pressure (Pcap) and subsequent edema formation. Relative intravascular volume reduction is due to edema formation the intravascular volume which triggers neurohumoral compensatory mechanisms. Which includes sympathetic nervous system (SNS), arginine vasopressin (AVP), and the renin angiotensin aldosterone system (RAAS), with

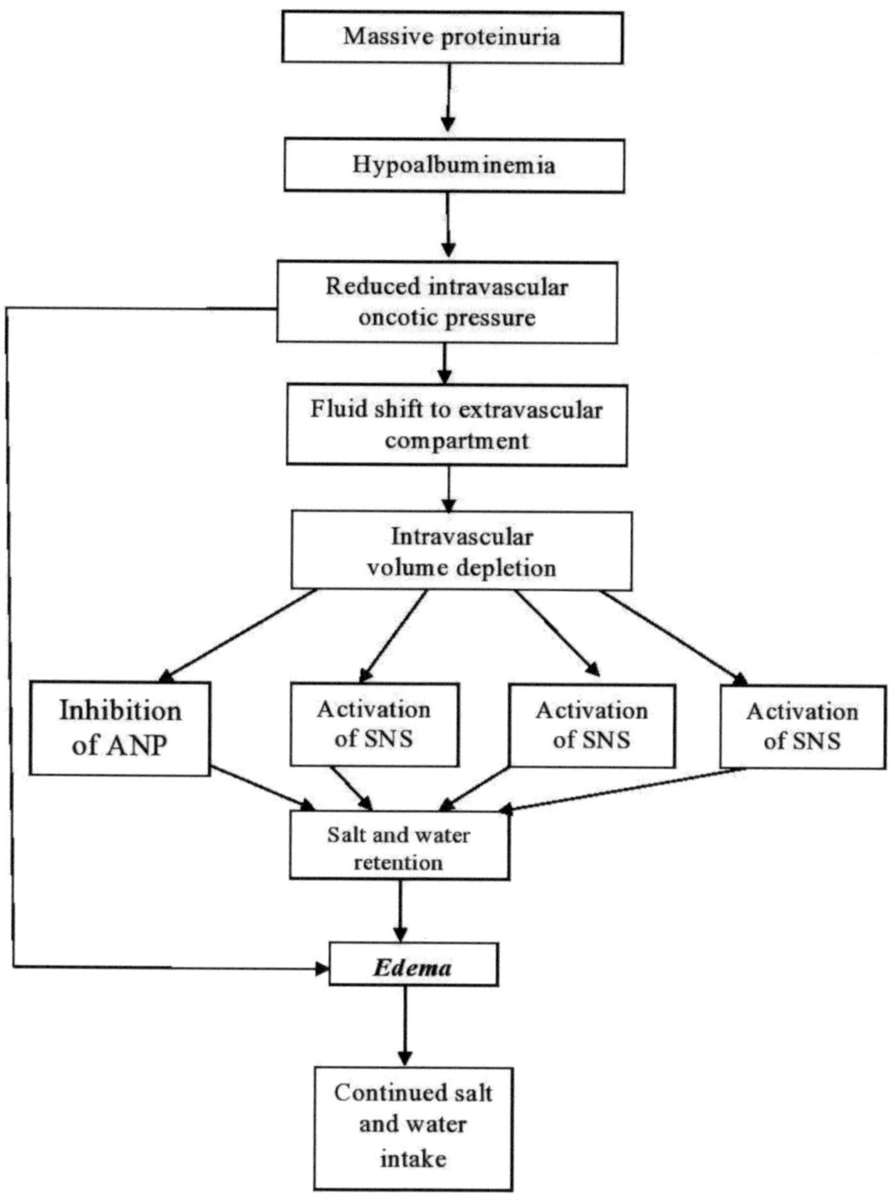

Figure 2.
Under fill hypothesis proposes the continuation of a reduced effective circulating blood volume in nephrotic syndrome. Pathophysiologic events leading to the formation of edema in nephrotic syndrome.

the net causes being sodium and water retention by the kidney. In the background of nephrotic syndrome, aortic arch, left ventricle, mechanoreceptors in the carotid sinus, and afferent arterioles in the glomeruli detect reduced pressure distension. This produce (1) SNS outflow increases from the central nervous system, (2) RAAS activation, and (3) nonosmotic release of AVP from the hypothalamus. These three changes lead to peripheral vasoconstriction (increased SNS and angiotensin II), sodium retention (angiotensin II, aldosterone, and increased SNS), and water retention.

As a result of these mechanisms, it is greatly accepted that patients with nephrotic syndrome have an excess of total body water and sodium. The condition of their intravascular volume is to some amount controvertible. Intravascular state in nephrotic is demonstrated by the following hypothesis: so-called overfill hypothesis and underfill hypothesis. The continuation of a reduced effective circulating blood volume in nephrotic syndrome is explained by underfill hypothesis (**Figure 2**). Due to activation of the RAAS with resultant of reduction in urinary sodium excretion and elevation of aldosterone levels, is most expectedly promoted by findings of low urine sodium in the presence of edema. The low urinary sodium [45] is due to reduction of atrial natriuretic peptide (ANP). Evidence, additionally for the underfill hypothesis includes betterment in sodium excretion with albumin infusion or head-out water immersion, and reduced cardiac output and increased vascular evaluated. It is possible that the overfilled state may be major in the chronic phase during which patients may have long-lasting sodium retention due to unrelenting low-grade hypoalbuminemia. But the underfilled state may be major in the acute setting in which excessive proteinuria causes rapid development of hypoalbuminemia and a gradual drop in plasma oncotic pressure.

Supposed to be intravascularly volume-expanded as different to degree-constricted, founding whether a child is underfilled versus overfilled can be clinically important in the edema in children with nephrotic syndrome may be different. Depends upon the below urinary estimations comparison with elevated plasma vasopressin, renin, norepinephrine, aldosterone levels they are Single group has support to estimate the relative urinary potassium excretion [UK/(UK + UNa and)] absolute excretion of sodium (FENa) to elucidate the distinction. Nephrotic patients who are with high urinary potassium excretion (>60%) and a low FENa (<1%) would be probable to have a low intravascular load [46].

5. Conclusion

Causes of nephrotic syndrome are also age reliant. The majority of the cases reported in the first 3 months of life is referred to as congenital nephrotic syndrome (CNS) and are because of genetic diseases. While there has been no efficient study of the etiology of nephrotic syndrome presenting in the rest of the first year of life (3–12 months), there are data telling that up to 40% of cases during this time may also be due to genetic causes. While it is extensively accepted that patients with nephrotic syndrome have an excess of total body sodium and water as a result of these remunerative mechanisms, the status of their intravascular volume is to some extent controversial. Nephrotic syndrome was a variety of disease processes with heavy proteinuria and hypoalbuminemia at its main symptoms. Although ongoing research hard work in the mechanism of disease, first-line therapy has stay over relatively unaffected for decades, and corticosteroids drugs are the basis of treatment Most children have MCNS, which come through a good prognosis; renal failure is uncommon in patients with MCNS. The manner of patients with nephrotic syndrome is changeable, but most patients will have periods of relapse and remission. Guidelines published by the American Academy of Pediatrics and the KDIGO can guide the pediatrician in the treatment of MCNS. There are alternative to corticosteroid therapy that has had

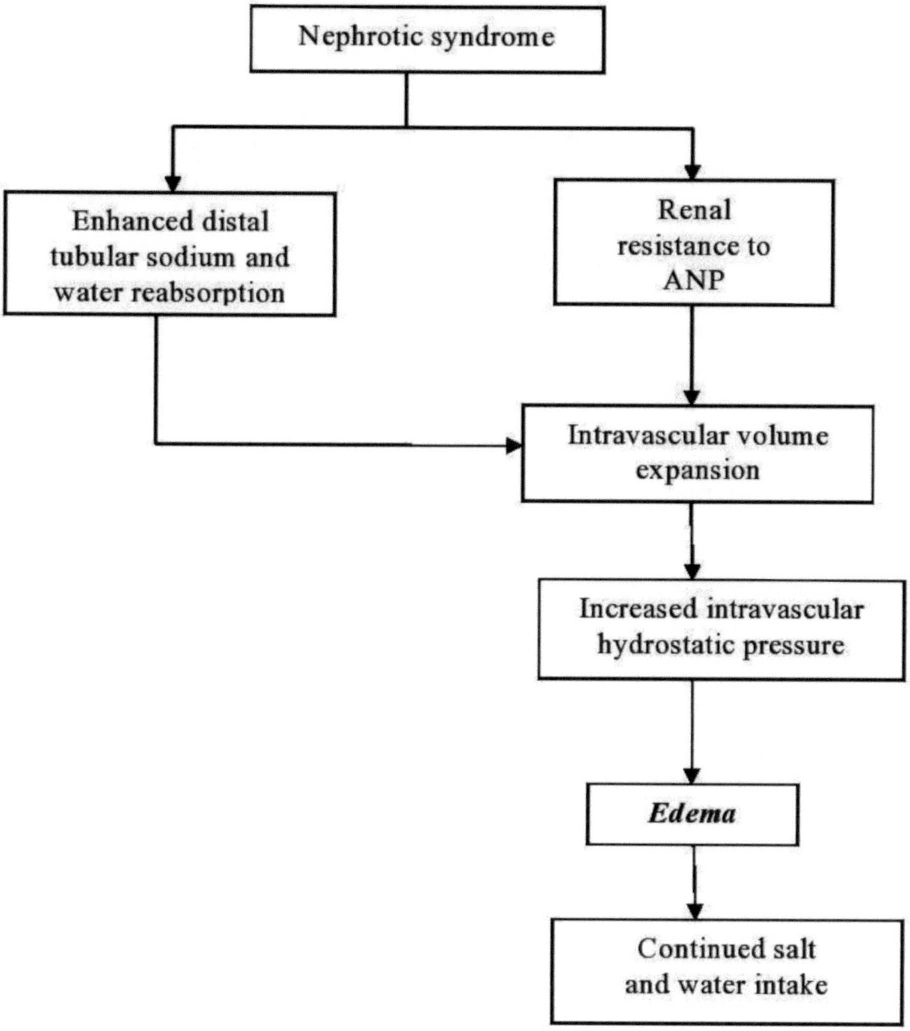

Figure 3.
Pathophysiologic events leading to the formation of edema in nephrotic syndrome according to the overfill hypothesis.

success in induction and/or maintenance of reduction, although findings are conflicting, necessitating additional multicenter trials to contrast these medications head to head. Hypotheses concerning the mechanisms of proteinuria and the possible association of glomerular structure to the nephrotic syndrome are discussed (**Figure 3**).

Conflict of interest

None declared.

Notes/Thanks/Other declarations

I am very much thankful to Dr. Manish Kumar Thimmaraju for his guidance, kind help and constant encouragement during progress of my work. I am also very thankful to my colleagues for the completion of this work.

Abbreviations

NS	nephrotic syndrome
CNS	congenital nephrotic syndrome
CNF	congenital nephrotic syndrome of the Finnish type
ESRD	end-stage renal disease
GBM	glomerular basement membrane
SRNS	steroid-resistant nephrotic syndrome
MPGN	membranoproliferative glomerulonephritis
FSGS	focal segmental glomerulosclerosis
MCNS	minimal-change nephrotic syndrome
RAAS	renin angiotensin aldosterone system
SNS	sympathetic nervous system
AVP	arginine vasopressin
GFB	glomerular filtration barrier
SRNS	steroid resistant nephrotic syndrome

Author details

Nagaraju Vallepu[1*], Saikiran Velpula[1], Bharath Kumar Dasari[1], Manish Kumar Thimmaraju[2], Sridhar Babu Gummadi[3], Neeraja Yelugam[1] and Supraja Jannu[1]

1 Department of Pharmacy Practice, Balaji Institute of Pharmaceutical Sciences, Warangal, Telangana, India

2 Department of Pharmaceutical Analysis, Balaji Institute of Pharmaceutical Sciences, Warangal, Telangana, India

3 Sri Shivani College of Pharmacy, Warangal, Telangana, India

*Address all correspondence to: vallepunagaraju99@gmail.com

References

[1] Cattran DC, Feehally J, Cook HT, Liu ZH, Fervenza FC, Mezzano SA, et al. Kidney disease: Improving global outcomes (KDIGO) glomerulonephritis work group. KDIGO clinical practice guideline for glomerulonephritis. Kidney International Supplements. 2012;**2**:139-274. DOI: 10.1038/kisup.2012.9

[2] Arneil GC. The nephrotic syndrome. Pediatric Clinics of North America. 1971;**18**(2):547-559

[3] Arneil GC, Lam CN. Long-term assessment of steroid therapy in childhood nephrosis. Lancet. 1966;**2**(7468):819-821

[4] Lenkkeri U et al. Structure of the gene for congenital nephritic syndrome of the Finnish type (NPHS1) and characterization of mutations. American Journal of Human Genetics. 1999;**64**(1):51-61

[5] Hinkes B et al. Genetic causes of nephrotic syndrome in the first year of life. American Pediatric Nephrology Meeting. Marburg; 2006

[6] Eddy AA, Symons JM. Nephrotic syndrome in childhood. Lancet. 2003;**362**(9384):629-639

[7] Gipson DS, Troost JP, Lafayette RA, et al. Complete remission in the nephrotic syndrome study network. Clinical Journal of the American Society of Nephrology. 2016;**11**:81-89

[8] Ruf RG et al. Patients with mutations in NPHS2 (podocin) do not respond to standard steroid treatment of nephrotic syndrome. Journal of the American Society of Nephrology. 2004;**15**(3):722-732

[9] Weber S et al. NPHS2 mutation analysis shows genetic heterogeneity of steroid-resistant nephrotic syndrome and low post-transplant recurrence. Kidney International. 2004;**66**(2):571-579

[10] Nash MA et al. The nephrotic syndrome. In: Edelmann CMJ, editor. *Pediatric Kidney Disease*. Boston: Little, Brown, and Company; 1992

[11] Srivastava T, Simon SD, Alon US. High incidence of focal segmental glomerulosclerosis in nephrotic syndrome of childhood. Pediatric Nephrology. 1999;**13**(1):13-18

[12] Ravani P, Rossi R, Bonanni A, et al. Rituximab in children with steroid-dependent nephrotic syndrome: A multicenter, open-label, noninferiority, randomized controlled trial. Journal of the American Society of Nephrology. 2015;**26**:2259-2266

[13] Coulthard MG. Oedema in kwashiorkor is caused by hypoalbuminaemia. Paediatrics and International Child Health. 2015;**35**:83-89

[14] Hogg RJ et al. Evaluation and management of proteinuria and nephrotic syndrome in children: Recommendations from a pediatric nephrology panel established at the National Kidney Foundation conference on proteinuria, albuminuria, risk, assessment, detection, and elimination (PARADE). Pediatrics. 2000;**105**(6):1242-1249

[15] McEnery PT, Strife CF. Nephrotic syndrome in childhood. Management and treatment in patients with minimal change disease, mesangial proliferation, or focal glomerulosclerosis. Pediatric Clinics of North America. 1982;**29**(4):875-894

[16] Bonilla-Felix M et al. Changing patterns in the histopathology of

idiopathic nephrotic syndrome in children. Kidney International. 1999;**55**(5):1885-1890

[17] Wong SN, Yu EC, Chan KW. Hepatitis B virus associated membranous glomerulonephritis in children—Experience in Hong Kong. Clinical Nephrology. 1993;**40**(3):142-147

[18] Bhimma R et al. Treatment of hepatitis B virus-associated nephropathy in black children. Pediatric Nephrology. 2002;**17**(6):393-399

[19] Filler G et al. Is there really an increase in non-minimal change nephrotic syndrome in children? American Journal of Kidney Diseases. 2003;**42**(6):1107-1113

[20] Smoyer WE, Mundel P. Regulation of podocyte structure during the development of nephrotic syndrome. Journal of Molecular Medicine. 1998;**76**(3-4):172-183

[21] White RH, Glasgow EF, Mills RJ. Clinicopathological study of nephrotic syndrome in childhood. Lancet. 1970;**1**(7661):1353-1359

[22] Brenner BM, Hostetter TH, Humes HD. Glomerular permselectivity: Barrier function based on discrimination of molecular size and charge. The American Journal of Physiology. 1978;**234**(6): F455-F460

[23] Kitano Y, Yoshikawa N, Nakamura H. Glomerular anionic sites in minimal change nephrotic syndrome and focal segmental glomerulosclerosis. Clinical Nephrology. 1993;**40**(4):199-204

[24] Carrie BJ, Salyer WR, Myers BD. Minimal change nephropathy: An electrochemical disorder of the glomerular membrane. The American Journal of Medicine. 1981;**70**(2):262-268

[25] Van den Born J et al. A monoclonal antibody against GBM heparin sulfate induces an acute selective proteinuria in rats. Kidney International. 1992;**41**(1):115-123

[26] ISKDC. Nephrotic syndrome in children: Prediction of histopathology from clinical and laboratory characteristics at time of diagnosis. Kidney International. 1978;**13**:159-165

[27] Shih NY et al. Congenital nephrotic syndrome in mice lacking CD2-associated protein. Science. 1999;**286**(5438):312-315

[28] Kaplan JM et al. Mutations in ACTN4, encoding alpha-actinin-4, cause familial focal segmental glomerulosclerosis. Nature Genetics. 2000;**24**(3):251-256

[29] Ruf RG et al. Prevalence of WT1 mutations in a large cohort of patients with steroid-resistant and steroid-sensitive nephrotic syndrome. Kidney International. 2004;**66**(2):564-570

[30] Winn MP et al. A mutation in the TRPC6 cation channel causes familial focal segmental glomerulosclerosis. Science. 2005;**308**(5729):1801-1804

[31] Mucha B et al. Members of the APN study group. Mutations in the Wilms' tumor 1 gene cause isolated steroid resistant nephritic syndrome and occur in exons 8 and 9. Pediatric Research. 2006;**59**(2):325-331

[32] Boute N et al. NPHS2, encoding the glomerular protein podocin, is mutated in autosomal recessive steroid-resistant nephrotic syndrome. Nature Genetics. 2000;**24**:349-354

[33] Barisoni L, Mundel P. Podocyte biology and the emerging understanding of podocyte diseases. American Journal of Nephrology. 2003;**23**(5):353-360

[34] Benzing T. Signaling at the slit diaphragm. Journal of the American Society of Nephrology. 2004;**15**(6):1382-1391

[35] Tryggvason K, Patrakka J, Wartiovaara J. Hereditary proteinuria syndromes and mechanisms of proteinuria. The New England Journal of Medicine. 2006;**354**(13):1387-1401

[36] Barbaux S et al. Donor splice-site mutations in WT1 are responsible for Frasier syndrome. Nature Genetics. 1997;**17**(4):467-470

[37] Morello R, Lee B. Insight into podocyte differentiation from the study of human genetic disease: Nail-patella syndrome and transcriptional regulation in podocytes. Pediatric Research. 2002;**51**(5):551-558

[38] Boerkoel CF et al. Mutant chromatin remodeling protein SMARCAL1 causes Schimke immuno-osseous dysplasia. Nature Genetics. 2002;**30**(2):215-220

[39] Zenker M et al. Human laminin beta2 deficiency causes congenital nephrosis with mesangial sclerosis and distinct eye abnormalities. Human Molecular Genetics. 2004;**13**(21):2625-2632

[40] Shalhoub RJ. Pathogenesis of lipoid nephrosis: A disorder of T-cell function. Lancet. 1974;**2**(7880): 556-560

[41] Kemper MJ, Wolf G, Muller-Wiefel DE. Transmission of glomerular permeability factor from a mother to her child. The New England Journal of Medicine. 2001;**344**(5):386-387

[42] Meyrier A. Mechanisms of disease: Focal segmental glomerulosclerosis. Nature Clinical Practice Nephrology. 2005;**1**(1):44-54

[43] Dantal J et al. Effect of plasma protein adsorption on protein excretion in kidney-transplant recipients with recurrent nephrotic syndrome. The New England Journal of Medicine. 1994;**330**(1):7-14

[44] Savin VJ et al. Circulating factor associated with increased glomerular permeability to albumin in recurrent focal segmental glomerulosclerosis. The New England Journal of Medicine. 1996;**334**(14):878-883

[45] Candiano G et al. Inhibition of renal permeability towards albumin: A new function of apolipoproteins with possible pathogenetic relevance in focal glomerulosclerosis. Electrophoresis. 2001;**22**(9):1819-1825

[46] Topaloglu R et al. T-cell subsets, interleukin-2 receptor expression and production of interleukin-2 in minimal change nephrotic syndrome. Pediatric Nephrology. 1994;**8**(6):649-652